INTERVENING IN ADOLESCENT PROBLEM BEHAVIOR

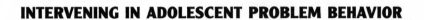

Intervening in Adolescent Problem Behavior

A FAMILY-CENTERED APPROACH

Thomas J. Dishion
Kate Kavanagh

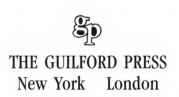

THE GUILFORD PRESS
New York   London

Printed in the United States of America

This book is printed on acid-free paper.

Last digit is print number: 9 8 7 6 5 4 3 2 1

Library of Congress Cataloging-in-Publication Data

Dishion, Thomas J., 1954–
    Intervening in adolescent problem behavior : a family-centered approach /
Thomas J. Dishion, Kate Kavanagh.
        p. cm.
Includes bibliographical references and index.
    ISBN 1-57230-874-5 (hc : alk. paper)
    1. Behavior therapy for teenagers. 2. Family psychotherapy I. Kavanagh, Kate.
II. Title.
    RJ505.B4D55 2003
    616.89′142′0835—dc21
                                                                2003002749

About the Authors

Thomas J. Dishion, PhD, is founder and Director of Research at the Child and Family Center, as well as Professor of Clinical Psychology, at the University of Oregon–Eugene. He specializes in research on the etiology and prevention of conduct problems and adolescent problem behavior, and has published over 70 empirical articles on screening, development, treatment, and prevention of child and adolescent problem behavior. He recently received an award from the Society for Research on Adolescence for research that had a significant impact on social policy affecting adolescents.

Kate Kavanagh, PhD, is a research associate at the Child and Family Center at the University of Oregon–Portland, as well as a consultant to the Portland Public School District's prevention office. Her research interests include understanding effective intervention and prevention practices for developing prosocial child and adolescent outcomes in families across the developmental continuum. She has published numerous scientific reports, and has presented at conferences and trainings throughout the United States.

Preface

This volume is intended as a comprehensive, science-based discussion of a family-centered approach to interventions for adolescent problem behavior. It is written for professionals working with adolescents and their families. Clinical, counseling, and school psychologists and social workers, as well as graduate students being trained to work with children and families, will find this material useful. In addition, program directors will find this volume particularly helpful for developing strategies to improve mental health and prevent substance use among young people within their communities.

In the approach described in this volume, we draw from the scientific literature on the development of problem behavior in adolescence, along with prevention and treatment literature on disruptive behavior in children and adolescents. Our perspective would be described as both ecological and family-centered. Put simply, parents *do* make a difference. Interventions that support parenting practices need to be tailored to the cultural background of the family and promote adaptive communication and collaboration with schools.

We understand that readers will find different areas of interest. Some will seek out the nuts and bolts of treatment, whereas others will focus more on the science and the larger perspective of which interventions are most likely to be effective. For the clinically oriented, we provide detailed discussion of empirically based intervention practices, often supported with brief clinical scenarios derived from our actual clinical experience; however, the key identifying character-

istics (name, gender, ethnicity) have been changed to ensure the
protection of confidentiality. We also refer the clinical reader to our
session-by-session intervention manual for working with parents
(Dishion et al., 2003).

For the scientist, data are reported throughout the volume, but
ample reference also is made to the scientific literature for further
follow-up. This work is based on over 15 years of work on the development of the Adolescent Transitions Program. The publications
from this study are available on the website of the Child and Family
Center at the University of Oregon (*http://cfc.uoregon.edu*).

Because dealing with pronouns is difficult, we have elected to al-
ternate between him and her and he and she throughout this book.
No implications are intended when using any pronoun. We attempt
only to maintain good grammar etiquette and impartiality between
male and female teens and parents.

We also refer to "parent" throughout the text. This term is used
synonymously for multiple parents, caregiver(s), or any person who
serves as a guardian(s) to teens.

Acknowledgments

We wish to acknowledge and thank the families who participated in the research leading to this volume. All the parents made a monumental effort to help their youngsters through the adolescent transition and placed the trust of their families in our hands. Their service to this project will have an impact on generations of parents to come, if we, as professionals, heed the data they provided us.

The work described in this volume began at the Oregon Social Learning Center. The database, intervention protocols, and assessment instruments build on 30 years of clinical and longitudinal research within the group, summarized in the writings of investigators Jerry Patterson, John Reid, Patti Chamberlain, Beverly Fagot, Marion Forgatch, Deborah Capaldi, Lew Bank, and Mike Stoolmiller. In addition, investigators from the Oregon Research Institute—Tony Biglan, Carol Metzler, and Blair Irvine—have helped in advancing both the assessment and intervention practices described here. We extend our appreciation to colleagues at both research centers for their encouragement, feedback, and collaboration.

We acknowledge the leadership at the National Institute on Drug Abuse—in particular, Drs. William Bukoski, Zilli Sloboda, Elizabeth Robertson, and, more recently, Aria Crump for their support of a program of research focusing on parenting and adolescent substance use.

We appreciate Ann Simas for her careful and patient work on the manuscript under the aegis of an uncertain time line and future, as is the case in the world of grant-funded research. The late Gene Brown is acknowledged for his scrupulous attention to detail in collecting and logging data from our Adolescent Transitions Program intervention trials. Finally, our science benefited from the ingenuity and attention to detail of Charlotte Winter in managing and analyzing the data over the course of this study.

Contents

PART I

An Ecological Overview

The ecological perspective provides a framework for understanding etiology, assessment-based decision making, case conceptualization, and designing context-sensitive interventions (Dishion & Stormshak, in press; Stormshak & Dishion, 2002). For example, one can think of an adolescent's behavior as "caused" by personal characteristics (e.g., anger, low self-esteem), friendships, a disrupted family, a high-risk neighborhood, and deviant models on television. From an ecological perspective, these are not incompatible hypotheses. Factors such as these are often linked together in a web of influences.

Our approach to research is to disentangle the various contextual influences into a comprehensive model that provides a guide to the design of interventions that is both effective and sensitive to the needs of families and adolescents within a variety of settings. As we argue throughout this volume, an ecological model of problem behavior is also a practical tool for designing assessment batteries and intervention strategies, and for formulating case conceptualizations.

In Chapter 1, we provide an overview of an ecological model for the development of adolescent problem behavior. Two interrelated features of the model are critical to understand: The model is developmental and family-centered. Chapter 2 provides an overview of how the ecological model is applied to the design of effective family-centered interventions that range from clinical treatment to prevention within schools and neighborhood communities.

1

A Family-Centered Model

The intervention and assessment practices described in this book are based on a family-centered model of adolescent problem behavior (Dishion & Patterson, 1999; Patterson, Reid, & Dishion, 1992). The model is derived from both basic research on social development and intervention science. In this chapter, we provide a look at the family-centered model as it applies to concerns for prevention and treatment.

We make two major points in this chapter. The first is that a developmental perspective is needed to understand the *function* of problem behavior from childhood through adolescence. An understanding of the function and ecology of adolescent problem behavior provides a foundation for designing effective interventions. The second point is that families in general, and parenting practices in particular, are critical to understanding, preventing, and treating adolescent problem behavior. Specifically, we refer to family management practices as the core set of parenting practices relevant to adolescent problem behavior.

DEVELOPMENTAL ISSUES

Problem behaviors in children and adolescents are those that (1) are experienced as troublesome by adults (such as parents and teachers) or (2) are known to disrupt normative social development. Generally, behaviors need to be judged relative to the age of the child. Although there are high stabilities in problem behavior in children over time (Loeber & Dishion, 1983; Olweus, 1979; Patterson, 1993), the form often changes from childhood to adolescence (Patterson, 1993).

When working with families, two developmental pathways must be considered in the case conceptualization (Moffitt, 1993; Patterson, 1993): (1) the "early-starter pathway," or children with a history of problem behavior (usually living in a disrupted environment), who escalate to more serious forms of antisocial behavior, including delinquency, drug use, and violence in early adolescence (Dishion, Capaldi, Spracklen, & Li, 1995; Pulkkinen, 1982); and (2) the "late-starter pathway," or youth with marginal adaptation to school and the peer group, who emerge as problematic in early to middle adolescence (Moffitt, 1993). Several researchers have emphasized that the form of problem behavior from early childhood may change in adolescence, but often the function remains the same (Dishion & Patterson, 1997; Patterson, 1993). A vast literature exists on the continuity of problem behavior over time (see Loeber, 1982; Loeber & Dishion, 1983; Olweus, 1979). Figure 1.1 provides an overview of the forms of problem behavior from early childhood through adolescence.

Age of onset for behavior problems is relevant to case conceptualization, primarily because of the increasing likelihood of academic and social skills deficits of youth with a history of problem behavior (Dishion, Loeber, Stouthamer-Loeber, & Patterson, 1984), peer sup-

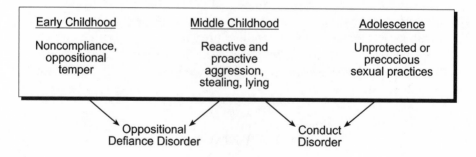

FIGURE 1.1. Developmental model of problem behavior from early childhood through adolescence.

port for problem behavior (Fergusson & Horwood, 2002), and the family's level of engagement in parenting (Patterson et al., 1992). Young adolescents who experiment with problem behavior, however, remain at risk for several negative life outcomes (Stattin & Magnusson, 1991), so intervention strategies must consider the needs of both groups simultaneously, inextricably linking prevention and treatment.

Problem behavior in early childhood occurs mostly in the context of the caregiving relationship. Parents report the problem behaviors of young children as noncompliance, defiance, aggression, and temper tantrums (Patterson, 1982). In more extreme cases, parents may complain about cruelty to pets, siblings, or peers in early childhood. The majority of such concerns have noncompliance at the core (Patterson, 1982). If these concerns are not addressed, then they may lead to more serious forms of antisocial behavior in middle childhood (Campbell, 1994; Shaw, Owens, Vondra, Keenan, & Winslow, 1996).

In middle childhood, the set of behaviors expands to include lying, stealing, and disruptive behavior, but still may include aggression and noncompliance. Considerable research has been done on the question of whether or not children "specialize" in specific forms of antisocial behavior such as stealing (i.e., covert) or overt forms of antisocial behavior (Loeber & Schmaling, 1985; Patterson et al., 1992). Although some children who are seen in clinical settings may specialize in stealing or aggressiveness (Patterson, 1982), those behaviors are generally highly correlated (Dishion, French, & Patterson, 1995).

The most promising differentiation in problem behavior to date is between proactive and reactive aggression (Dodge, 1991; Dodge & Coie, 1987; Poulin, Dishion, & Burraston, 2001; Pulkkinen, 1996; Vitaro, Gendreau, Tremblay, & Oligny, 1998). Reactive aggression describes a child's tendency to respond emotionally to peer provocations with aggression. Proactive aggression, alternatively, often involves planned attacks on a peer, usually in the company of other peers. Bullying is a form of proactive aggression (Hawkins, Pepler, & Craig, 2001; Olweus, 1991). The switch into proactive aggression reflects a tendency to engage in antisocial behavior with peers (Poulin & Boivin, 2000). Children who are proactively aggressive may engage in other, "covert" antisocial behaviors such as lying and stealing (Loeber & Schmaling, 1985). We see these covert forms of behavior emerge in early adolescence simultaneously with increased involvement with the deviant peer group (Dishion, Patterson, Stoolmiller, & Skinner, 1991).

The form of problem behavior in middle childhood varies for boys and girls (Cairns & Cairns, 1984). Clearly, by this age, we are seeing more signs of overt aggression in boys and relational aggression in girls (Crick, 1996; Grotpeter & Crick, 1996). Relational aggression describes psychological attacks, such as ostracism and gossip. Engagement in these activities appears linked to poor social and emotional adjustment in girls (Crick, 1996). As an interesting aside, parents are often less aware of girls' relational aggression, because it occurs at school in the company of friends. Given that teachers also may be less aware, the research suggests that it may be more difficult to detect the early signs of problem behavior and future adjustment difficulties of girls.

The link between antisocial behavior in middle childhood and the emergence of new problem behavior in adolescence is quite strong (Cairns, Cairns, Neckerman, Ferguson, & Gariepy, 1989; Loeber, 1982; Loeber & Dishion, 1983; Patterson, 1993). In both girls and boys, we see the use of substances (Dishion, Capaldi, & Yoerger, 1999), a pull away from parental supervision (Stoolmiller, 1990), and, eventually, sexual precocity (Capaldi, Crosby, & Stoolmiller, 1996; Rosenbaum & Kandel, 1990). Without a doubt, the adolescent performance of these problem behaviors is more than an irritation for parents. Early-onset substance use, for instance, predicts substance abuse in young adults (Dishion & Owen, 2002; Kandel, Davies, Karus, & Yamaguchi, 1986; Newcomb & Bentler, 1988; Robins & Przybeck, 1985; Yamaguchi & Kandel, 1985).

It is tempting to develop separate treatment programs for problem behaviors such as conduct disorders, substance use, and even depression. In adolescence, many of these behaviors co-occur (Jessor & Jessor, 1977; Metzler, Noell, & Biglan, 1992). Although these behaviors do correlate in a problem behavior syndrome, we argue that it is critical to consider the function of the behavior when designing intervention and treatment programs (Dishion & Patterson, 1997), as well as developmental sequencing (Loeber, 1988). For instance, some adolescents may increase their substance use as a function of an intervention delivered in peer groups, but a similar intervention strategy may work for other, less socially oriented adolescents, such as those who are purely depressed (e.g., Lewinsohn & Clark, 1990).

A variety of other adjustment difficulties may co-occur with adolescent problem behavior. When this is the case, it is often true that interventions addressing the problem behavior form the foundation of a long-term intervention solution. For instance, attention deficits form the substrate for the developmental sequencing described earlier. Children with attention deficit disorder have difficulty regulating behavior and emotion, and are the most vulnerable to the development of behavior problems (Barkley, Edwards, Laneri, Fletcher, & Metevia, 2001; Rothbart & Bates, 1998).

Most research indicates that attention deficits are often secondary to the problem behavior, with respect to the long-term outcomes, which suggests that interventions address both the problem behavior and the secondary symptoms (Chilcoat & Breslau, 1999; Hinshaw, 1987; Magnusson, 1988). This principle applies to other, co-occurring adjustment difficulties as well (e.g., depression, peer rejection, and learning difficulties). Generally speaking, we see comorbidity as a sign of clinical severity. For example, adolescents who are comorbid on depression and conduct problems have the most conflictual families (Granic & Lamey, 2002) and peer deviance (Dishion, 2000), compared to adolescents who show only problem behavior.

FUNCTIONALISM

Central to an ecological approach to intervention and developmental science is a functional understanding of adaptation (Dishion & Stormshak, in press). Learning theory led to the design of interventions that focus on reinforcement contingencies for positive and negative behaviors in settings such as the home and the school. Often, in the case of child problem behaviors, changing the contingencies of a behavior reduces its occurrence (Patterson, 1982). This concern with the function of a behavior in social interactions has been helpful in understanding and changing antisocial behavior in families (Dishion & Patterson, 1999), and reducing problem behavior in schools (Sugai, Horner, & Sprague, 1999).

In parent–child interactions, coercive processes are involved in the early emergence of aggressive behavior (Gardner, 1992; Snyder, Edwards, McGraw, Kilgore, & Holton, 1994) and later, more serious antisocial behavior (Patterson et al., 1992). Coercion also seems to be a common yet powerful organizing principle in many interpersonal relationships, such as unhappy marriages (Gottman, 1998) and distressed parent–adolescent relationships (Forgatch & Stoolmiller, 1994; Prinz, Foster, Kent, & O'Leary, 1979; Robin & Foster, 1989).

The basic process that underlies the disruptive effect of coercive interactions on relationships appears to be escape conditioning (Patterson, 1982). Figure 1.2 illustrates the escape conditioning mechanism underlying parent–adolescent coercion.

Within an escalating cycle of conflict, the parent reacts emotionally to a problem behavior. Emotional overreactions to adolescent problem behavior can often make the situation worse. For instance, a parent may "ground" her son for 2 months in response to his coming home 1 hour late. A week of complaining by the disgruntled teenager may lead to the parent eventually "giving up." The cycle, especially if repeated, leads to the gradual defeat of the adult caregiving system, as well as disaffected family relationships. The twofold cost of the coercion cycle, then, is that the teenager will be less likely to take the parent seriously, and the parent avoids a leadership role in the family.

In passing, it is important to note that the coercion cycle can underlie a variety of teenage difficulties, including sulking, depressed affect, restrictive eating, arguing, and so forth. The key is not so much the behavior content, but the functional process between the parent and the adolescent, as described earlier. For example, depressive affect can *function* to reduce parent–child conflict (e.g., Hops, Sherman, & Biglan, 1990).

Parents may sense a further loss of control when teenagers be-

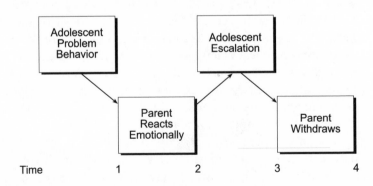

FIGURE 1.2. The escape conditioning mechanism underlying parent–adolescent coercion.

come emotionally invested in friendships and dating. Puberty, media, schools, and neighborhoods combine to account for the enormous influence of peers at this stage of life (Dishion, Poulin, & Medici Skaggs, 2000). This is especially true for youth with a history of problem behavior, family disruptions, and marginalizing school experiences. Youth with early-starting problem behavior tend to aggregate into high-risk peer groups as early as middle school (Dishion et al., 1991).

Beginning in early childhood, we find that aggressive children affiliate with other aggressive children (Snyder, West, Stockemer, Givens, & Almquist-Parks, 1996). The tendency of the problem child to affiliate with other antisocial children increases through middle childhood (Cairns, Perrin, & Cairns, 1985) and escalates in adolescence. The reason adolescent friendships are so important is that some are organized around deviance. We studied hundreds of adolescent friendships and have been able to identify a "deviant friendship process" that predicts escalating cycles of drug use (Dishion, Capaldi, et al., 1995), delinquency (Dishion, Spracklen, Andrews, & Patterson, 1996), and violence (Dishion, Eddy, Haas, Li, & Spracklen, 1997).

Adolescents can develop a style of connecting with other adolescents that virtually guarantees their friends will reinforce problem behavior in the future: that is, if not for breaking the rules and engaging in problem behavior, the adolescent friends would have nothing in common on which to base friendship. For this reason, the friendships are powerful and difficult to change once in place. The matching law (Conger et al., 1992; Hernstein, 1961; McDowell, 1988) accounts for such functional dynamics in relationships: The relative rate of reinforcement for deviant talk accounts for the overall rates within the friendship, which in turn, predict escalations in problem behavior in the future.

Understanding the dynamics of deviant friendships is much more than an academic enterprise. We inadvertently discovered that aggregating high-risk young adolescents into group interventions actually leads to *increases* in their substance use and delinquent behavior at school (Dishion & Andrews, 1995).

When we first discovered this negative effect for peer aggregation (see Chapter 10 for more detail), we looked for other examples of similar findings in the literature, concerned that our finding was a statistical aberration. What we encountered was difficulty in finding evidence for *negative* effects because of the "file drawer" problem (Dawes, 1994). Psychologists do not typically publish null effects, let alone *mention* negative effects. Despite this bias, reviews of the literature on interventions for delinquent youth revealed that 29% had negative effects (Lipsey, 1992).

Our attention quickly focused on the work of Joan McCord, who repeatedly published the negative effects associated with a delinquency prevention experiment conducted before the Great Depression (McCord, 1979, 1992). In one of the most carefully conducted prevention experiments of our time, McCord found 30-year negative effects associated with involvement in the intervention.

McCord recently reanalyzed the Cambridge–Somerville data and found that it was primarily the aggregation into summer camps that accounted for the 30-year negative effects. If an "experimental" youth attended two consecutive summer camps, the odds ratio of a 30-year negative life outcome (compared to his carefully matched control) was 10:1 (Dishion, McCord, & Poulin, 1999).

Because most social programs that aggregate high-risk children probably provide less supervision than a clinical outcome study, we suggest that these findings may present a conservative picture of the potential risk associated with similar intervention strategies. These data together provide a strong message: Peer deviancy training is to be taken seriously in considering the intervention needs of adolescents (Dishion, McCord, et al., 1999).

It would be a mistake to conclude from such data that because of such pronounced and strong effects of peers in adolescence, adults are relatively unimportant. Consider that adults structured the high-risk peer groups that led to the iatrogenic effect. We hope that, in the future, community programs and leaders will eliminate programs that inadvertently encourage escalations in problem behavior. This is a formidable task given that most educational and juvenile justice interventions, for both cost and systemic reasons, involve aggregation of high-risk youth.

The functional emphasis within an ecological perspective has led to understanding another dynamic that is relevant to coercion and deviancy training. This involves the negative influence of siblings on social development. A reoccurring finding in the literature on adolescent problem behavior is that a small percentage of families produce a disproportionately large percentage of the crime in any given community (e.g., Farrington [1991] reports that 6% of families produce about 48% of the criminal acts within a community).

We believe there are two reasons for this finding. One is that some parents may actually encourage antisocial behavior, therefore directly contributing to the early emergence of problem behavior (Dishion, Bullock, & Owen, 2002). The other is that young adolescents and their siblings actively encourage deviance and collude to undermine adult supervision and guidance.

We directly observed 50 families; half were deemed as high risk in middle school by teacher ratings, and half were noted as successful by virtue of grades and good conduct (Bullock & Dishion, 2002). As expected, we directly observed siblings colluding to undermine parental attempts to guide and manage their behavior in problem-solving tasks we structured (Bullock & Dishion, 2003). Often, parents' efforts to guide and lead were obfuscated by the alternative goals of the "sibling system." This dynamic speaks to a problem that has long troubled family therapists—how to get parents to serve an executive function in families (Minuchin & Fishman, 1981; Szapocznik, Kurtines, & Fernandez, 1980).

FAMILY MANAGEMENT

Placing parents in the central role in socialization is not entirely based on correlational and longitudinal data. Simple pragmatism suggests that parents are the key agents of change within a system designed to socialize youth. To this end, it is important to consider the ecology of parenting.

Reviews of the literature concur that family management reduces coercive family interactions (Dishion, Burraston, & Li, 2002; Forgatch, 1991; Patterson et al., 1992), the likelihood of deviant peer involvement and deviancy training (Dishion, Spracklen, Andrews, & Patterson, 1996; Patterson & Dishion, 1985), and sibling collusion (Bullock & Dishion, 2002). In this sense, we conceptualize family management as a protective factor in adolescence. However, little research has formally tested this hypothesis in the conventional statistical framework, with the notable exception of the pioneering research by Wilson (1980). His research indicated that in high-crime areas in inner-city London, parental supervision was a key protective factor for preventing delinquency.

In general, we see parenting as both directly and indirectly related to adolescent adjustment. In particular, parenting is a joint outcome of three embedded processes (Dishion & McMahon, 1998): (1) having a positive relationship with an adolescent; (2) being effective in managing behavior; and (3) monitoring and attending to behavior. During adolescence, monitoring tends to wane in families and therefore deserves special clinical attention. The direct relationship is documented in various studies showing that poor parental monitoring predicts early substance use (Baumrind, 1985; Dishion & Loeber, 1985). Parental monitoring is also indirectly related to substance use via its impact on time spent with peers. Children who are not well monitored tend to wander about the community, freely selecting places that involve drug use and other delinquent activities (Patterson & Dishion, 1985; Stoolmiller, 1994).

Effective parenting may take on a variety of forms depending on the culture, community context, or constellation of the family. The vast majority of parents are invested in their children's success and good health. As children mature, there is a natural tension that leads to increasing levels of independence and autonomy (Dishion et al., 2000; Granic, Dishion, & Hollenstein, 2003). Although parenting in early and middle childhood sets the stage, continued parental support and positive family management can help reduce risk and provide protection during the adolescent transition. In Figure 1.3, we provide an overview of how we see parenting interact with other sources of influence in the social and emotional development of adolescents.

As noted in Figure 1.3, family management is seen as influencing the peer and sibling environment and adolescent adjustment. Clearly, adolescents can impact the parents' selection of parenting strategies (firm vs. lax) by virtue of the seriousness of their problem behavior or the community context. A parent of an adolescent may be strict about activities after curfew in a community plagued with high violence or police monitoring. Working with these families requires knowledge and sensitivity about community setting, appreciation of cultural differences in effective parenting, and flexibility with respect to a menu of intervention activities.

Note that, in Figure 1.3, we include biological characteristics of

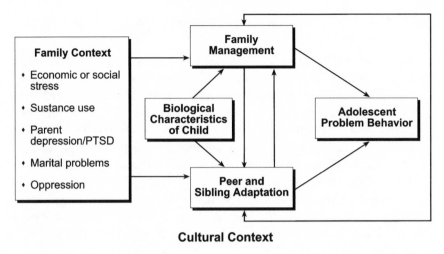

FIGURE 1.3. Parental interaction with other sources of influence in the social and emotional development of adolescents.

the child as not having a direct effect on adolescent problem behavior except by virtue of disrupted family environments, or by deviant peer influences. Clearly, factors such as the child's gender (Moffitt, Caspi, Rutter, & Silva, 2001), attention (Rothbart, Posner, & Hershey, 1995), and other genetically transmitted characteristics (Rhee & Waldman, 2002) are influential within the socialization process. We propose, however, that the most important influence of the child's temperament is the potential to disrupt family management or to evoke negative peer influences.

Research on parenting clarifies that it is what parents do, and not their history, that has the most influence on children's protection and risk. Parents who have insight about their own past, and who have acquired parenting skills to respond competently, are less likely to perpetuate pathology across generations (Egeland & Susman-Stillman, 1996; Forgatch, 1991). Researchers are beginning to converge on a set of parenting practices that are relevant to positive youth development: relationship building, limit-setting, positive reinforcement, monitoring, and conflict resolution (Hawkins, Catalano, & Miller, 1992; Patterson et al., 1992). It is important to note, however, that the style and emphasis on these components of family management vary by family ethnicity (Dishion & Bullock, 2001).

THE ECOLOGY OF PARENTING

The model we propose incorporates the reality that circumstances can disrupt parenting, and that peers often have a powerful influence. Sometimes the disruption in family management results from relationship changes (i.e., divorce or remarriage). Other times, the parents' behavior and adjustment interferes with family management. For instance, parental substance use is clearly a risk factor for early adolescent drug use and may undermine parental ability to establish abstinence norms for children (Chassin, Presson, Sherman, Montello, & McGrew, 1986). Similarly, economic stress, job loss (Conger et al., 1992; Elder, Van Nguyen, & Caspi, 1985), or long-standing disadvantage (McLoyd, 1990) can disrupt parenting and ultimately add to potential risk. Family management can buffer the effects of such stress, although, under some circumstances, this may require Herculean efforts. Eventually, social contexts that are high in poverty, oppression, unemployment, and crime will undermine all but a few families.

Cultural stress occurs in a variety of forms and affects a growing number of families. It is difficult for parents to bridge the gap between two cultural worlds. Although this challenge may be especially evident in Hispanic families (Szapocznik et al., 1980), the same issues are equally present in other cultural groups as well. Acculturation level can have a disruptive impact on parenting. Interventions that provide support (bicultural training) for parents under these stressful circumstances are known to improve family functioning and positive outcomes in children (Szapocznik et al., 1997).

A history of oppression can also disrupt cultural strengths in parenting. Consider the effect of colonization on American Indian families, particularly the practice of forcibly removing children from families and sending them to distant boarding schools, where English and European culture was imposed (Duran & Duran, 1995). These practices, as well as other events that have attacked the integrity and pride of indigenous peoples around the world, certainly undermine the performance of parenting practices, engineered carefully over thousands of years.

Other sources of family disruption come from within. A growing number of families experience the disruption of divorce and remarriage. These events are not trivial in the lives of children. Family management is clearly a protective factor in the context of divorce

(Forgatch, Patterson, & Skinner, 1988). How parents handle conflict and their children's best interests is the key factor in explaining why some children remain healthy and successful in the face of serious problems (Buchanan, Maccoby, & Dornbusch, 1991; Maccoby, Depner, & Mnookin, 1990). The number of remarriage transitions is linearly related to the level of maladjustment, including the use of drugs in childhood and early adolescence. However, the use of positive family management practices can dramatically reduce that risk (Capaldi & Patterson, 1991).

The evidence is clear that the ecology of parenting is relevant to child adjustment. We propose that family management practices, under many circumstances, can serve as a protective factor in the face of adverse, risky environments. Given this protective role, parenting practices are a prime target for intervention programs.

FAMILY INTERVENTIONS WORK

We find it helpful to make a distinction between interventions that support existing parenting competencies and those that target risk factors or family dysfunction. As discussed in Chapter 3, these two levels of intervention can be integrated. The bulk of the more rigorous research involving control groups and random assignment focuses on interventions that target risk and dysfunction (notable exception, Kumpfer, Molgaard, & Spoth, 1996).

Research indicates that interventions aimed at improving parenting practices result in the reduction of risk factors. Figure 1.4 summarizes the findings on the effectiveness of family-based interventions. These conclusions are based on the assiduous efforts of the top intervention scientists.

The effectiveness of intervention in early childhood has implications for the prevention of antisocial behavior in middle childhood and, ultimately, in adolescence. Researchers have found that parenting interventions are effective in reducing behavior problems in early childhood (Dadds, Spence, Holland, Barrett, & Lacrens, 1997; Webster-Stratton, 1984, 1990). Webster-Stratton showed that parenting groups that focus on providing support and skills development for young families produce marked improvements in observed parent–child interactions and teacher ratings of problems in preschool. Additionally, these positive effects persisted for at least 3

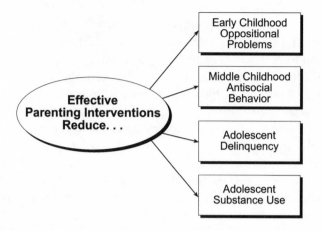

FIGURE 1.4. The effectiveness of family-based interventions.

years after the intervention. A critical piece of the Webster-Stratton program is the development of videotaped examples of positive parenting practices. These tapes are so useful to parents that change was observed in children's behavior as a function of the videotapes, without the help of therapists (Webster-Stratton, Kolpacoff, & Hollingsworth, 1988). However, in general, mothers preferred to use the videotapes in leader-guided parent training groups.

Antisocial and aggressive behavior in childhood is a major predictor of adolescent drug use (Kellam, Brown, Rubin, & Ensminger, 1983). Interventions that target parenting practices are the most promising for reducing antisocial behavior in middle childhood (Dumas, 1989; Kazdin, 1993; Patterson, Dishion, & Chamberlain, 1993). The evidence is extensive and impressive. Patterson (1974) found that parent training interventions were effective in reducing antisocial behavior in the home and at school. Johnson and Christensen (1975) revealed that the impact of parent training was evidenced in parent perceptions, direct observations in the home, and brief telephone interviews. It is important to note that parents are satisfied with parent training (McMahon, Tiedemann, Forehand, & Griest, 1993).

An advantage of family-based interventions is that the benefits accrue for all family members. For example, Arnold, Levine, and Patterson (1975) documented that parent training produced statistically reliable changes in the behavior of the siblings of the referred child. This finding is particularly relevant when considering that drug abuse and serious delinquency tends to run in families.

A frequent assumption is that interventions in adolescence are a waste of time and resources, because prevention is only possible if there is intervention at younger years. The data suggest, however, that this simply is not true. Intervention during adolescence is critical within an overall prevention strategy, with respect to reducing problem behaviors. Directly and indirectly, these interventions can have a positive effect on the next generation, for example, simply by reducing the likelihood of teenage parenting or spacing children in young families (Olds, 2002).

Harm reduction is an explicit goal of intervention in the adolescent phase of development. If interventions reduce the escalating cycle of drug abuse, delinquency, sexual precocity, or extensive incarceration, it is possible that negative outcomes in early adulthood can be prevented. From this perspective, interventions that reduce risk and promote adaptation at one stage promote success in the next developmental transition (Dishion & Kavanagh, 2002).

Results of outcome studies indicate that family-centered interventions during adolescence are effective in reducing current problem behavior and future risk (Alexander & Parsons, 1973; Bank, Marlowe, Reid, Patterson, & Weinrott, 1991; Henggeler, Melton, & Smith, 1992; Henggeler et al., 1986). Relevant to this discussion, the data suggest that interventions promoting positive family management reduce adolescent substance use (Bry & Canby, 1986; Bry, McKeon, & Pardina, 1982; Friedman, 1989; Huey, Henggeler, Brondino, & Pickrel, 2000; Lewis, Piercy, Sprendle, & Trepper, 1990; Schmidt, Liddle, & Dakof, 1996). As discussed in Chapter 10, our findings on the effectiveness of family-centered interventions build on this important body of research.

SUMMARY

The etiology of problem behavior is not a mysterious accumulation of risk factors. Both the developmental and intervention data support a focus on family management as central to the risk process leading to adolescent problem behavior. The family-centered model incorporates all levels of influence, including biology, parenting, peers, and the ecology. The emphasis on family management offers an intervention focus. This model, however, does not suggest that parents are to blame for problem behavior (Harris, 1995), but rather that parenting is an important part of the solution. In this sense, intervention strategies that promote family management and adult involvement are critical for the long-term effectiveness of prevention.

In the next chapter, we turn our attention to an intervention framework that is helpful for considering how a focus on family management is both realistic and potentially helpful.

2

The ATP Multilevel Intervention Strategy

SOME HISTORY

About 15 years ago, we set out to design a prevention strategy based on a developmental model of adolescent problem behavior (Dishion, Reid, & Patterson, 1988). The set of interventions and materials that resulted from that effort is referred to as the Adolescent Transitions Program (ATP). The program has grown as a function of a series of intervention studies, both our own and those of others.

We began by using a conventional psychoeducational intervention model, relying on cognitive behavioral theories of behavior change. Based on developmental research on problem behavior (e.g., Dishion & Loeber, 1985; Loeber & Dishion, 1983; Patterson & Dishion, 1985), we targeted family management practices and deviant peer influences.

The groups were offered to self-identified, high-risk adolescents and their families as an outpatient service (Dishion et al., 1988). Families were randomly assigned to one of four intervention conditions and well paid for participating in the research. The findings taught us a great deal about the basic principles of intervening with high-risk adolescents and their families. For instance, we learned that unanticipated side effects can be more powerful than the intervention effects we presume (Dishion & Andrews, 1995).

Based on our findings, we began to implement the program within the school setting (Dishion, Andrews, Kavanagh, & Soberman, 1996). We were surprised at the heterogeneity of the risk population, as identified in schools, which ranged from adolescents just beginning to engage in problem behavior to those with a long developmental history (the early starters). It was alarming to us that many of the early-starting adolescents had never had contact with mental health services, in general, and parenting intervention services, in particular. In general, it seems to be true that conduct disordered adolescents infrequently have contact with any kind of mental health service, let alone an empirically supported intervention (Stouthamer-Loeber, Loeber, Van Kammen, & Zhiang, 1995).

Finally, after years of running parent groups in schools, our intervention model broadened even further. We found ourselves spending time consulting with school personnel on strategies for working more constructively with students and their families. These school "system" efforts seemed important to the effectiveness of interventions; therefore, we incorporated them into our model (Dishion, Andrews, et al., 1996).

When we began to collaborate with schools in our Oregon community to implement ATP outside our grant research, we learned other lessons. For example, as school personnel often predicted, it was difficult to get high-risk parents to attend our 12-session parent groups. In one project, only 2 out of 50 identified parents showed up to the group. We concluded, after several such experiences, that we needed to expand the range of parent interventions to enhance the potential to engage parents in the school environment. We broadened the "menu" of intervention activities even further to have an impact on the parenting practices.

To broaden the scope of ATP, we moved in two directions. First, we designed a relatively brief intervention that incorporated advancements in motivational interviewing (Miller & Rollnick, 2002). We referred to our motivational intervention as the Family Check-Up (FCU). Initial data suggested promising results for this brief intervention as a change strategy (Rao, 1998). The second direction we took was to develop an intervention that permeated the school ecology. The goal of this "universal" intervention was to reach parents through a variety of school venues, in order to increase the potential of engagement and support.

Although the revisions to ATP have been data-based, they came to the research team with growing pains. The data demanded a review of our basic assumptions about the nature of clinical psychology and the change process, for instance, the assumption that the more sessions a parent engaged in, the more change could be expected. We did not find this "dose–response" relationship in either our individual family therapy model (Weber, 1998) or our group interventions with parents (see Chapter 10). Another assumption is that interventions should be delivered in a manual-like format, to ensure fidelity in implementation. Although a manual was useful for ensuring a sufficient level of fidelity in implementing our ATP intervention program, rigidly adhering to it was associated with *less* change in our parent groups (see Dishion et al., 2003).

Yet another example of a questionable assumption was that, as clinical psychologists, the primary venue of our work was to conduct "sessions" with parents or families in the mental health clinic. Like other investigators (e.g., Henggeler, Schoenwald, Borduin, Rowland, & Cunningham, 1998; Szapocznik & Kurtines, 1989), we found that in order to be effective, we had to leave the clinic and visit families in their homes, work with them in schools, and explore other strategies for affecting parenting practices.

Looking back at the changes with a perspective that the data forced on us, we now see that we were moving from a "medical" model of change to what we now call an ecological model (Stormshak & Dishion, 2002). The shift is critical to discuss at the outset of this volume, because it provides the rationale for designing an intervention program that is broader in focus and scope than the typical mental health treatment program. We begin by discussing the ATP model within the context of the "ecological cube," a framework originally proposed for the conceptualization and design of counseling services (Morrill, Oetting, & Hurst, 1974).

THE ECOLOGICAL CUBE

The ecological cube in Figure 2.1 summarizes the three dimensions of interventions now represented in our ATP model. The first issue is to consider the target of the intervention. In some ways, this can be surmised from developmental research. For example, in responding to

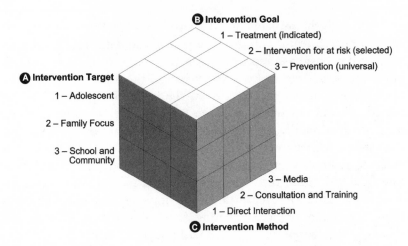

FIGURE 2.1. The ecological framework for intervention.

adolescent problem behavior, our developmental and intervention research suggests that interventions are most effective if they are
family-centered. However, as we all know, parents are not always immediately available. In fact, sometimes it is helpful to work directly
with the adolescent and be sensitive to what can often be delicate
family dynamics. In this way, every intervention target on the ecological cube focuses on directly or indirectly supporting family management.

The second dimension (i.e., intervention goal) suggests the need
to design interventions that address the developmental history of the
problem. Applied to problem behavior, the therapist must differenti-
ate interventions that address the needs of early versus late starters,
for example.

The third issue to be considered is the intervention method. In
our ATP model, the intervention method may involve direct interactions with parents and adolescents, consultation and training of
school personnel, or the use of didactic or inspirational media.

The ATP model is designed to include the entire cube. To accomplish a comprehensive intervention model such as ATP, we found that
it is necessary to blur the boundaries between the traditional professional roles of counseling and clinical psychology (Dishion & Stormshak, in press). For example, to prevent the emergence of problems in

a 13-year-old girl, it may be necessary to provide brief counseling services to her parents concerning the expected changes they may experience related to puberty or the girl's move to high school. This kind of counseling is provided in the FCU.

In addition to being comprehensive, other features of an ecological framework deserve mention, by way of introduction, that are critical for understanding how a comprehensive approach, such as ATP, might make a difference in improving outcomes in children at the community level.

PUBLIC HEALTH PERSPECTIVE

An implicit goal of helping professionals in mental health is to reduce the prevalence of psychopathology in children and families. However, if we design interventions that are limited in any dimension of the ecological cube, then our efforts are unlikely to have such a public health impact. To this extent, ATP is designed to address comprehensively the full range of families within a community, providing a multilevel strategy that links prevention with treatment. Although universal interventions may have only a small effect for an individual family, the small effect, because it reaches so many families, can add to a rather large effect for the community (Biglan, 1995; Kellam, 1990). Attending only to the needs of the 5% of families who are the most serious (e.g., Chamberlain & Reid, 1998; Henggeler et al., 1998) neglects families who are potentially moving into the high-risk range. In addition, universal interventions can mobilize community strengths that reduce conditions that exacerbate problem behavior among those most at risk. The ATP has a universal component that links with the selected and indicated interventions to reinforce intervention activities at all levels.

SERVICE DELIVERY SYSTEMS

Hoagwood and Koretz (1996) suggested that the public health would be benefited most if we focused the design of our interventions to fit within existing service delivery systems, especially those that affect large numbers of children and families.

In the United States, the vast majority of children up to the age of 13–14 attend school. Moreover, schools serve as convenient meeting places for deviant peer groups (Dishion, Duncan, Eddy, Fagot, & Fetrow, 1994; Kellam, 1990; Rutter, 1985). Attending to the school environment, as well as to family dynamics, is necessary to effect comprehensive reductions in children's problem behavior (Patterson, 1974). In addition, there is a gross mismatch between the needs of adolescents and the operation of the middle school setting (Eccles, Lord, & Roeser, 1995). Preventive intervention programs, therefore, need to "consider schools as potential sites for service delivery, as well as potential objects of intervention activity" (Trickett & Birman, 1989, p. 361).

CENTRALITY OF ASSESSMENT

Clinical judgments are fallible (Dawes, 1994). A third feature of the ecological approach is that case conceptualizations and interventions are based on structured assessments. For these assessments to be useful, it is necessary to assess the behavior of the child across settings (e.g., home and school), family interaction and management processes, and peer influences, as well as other cultural and community factors.

Case conceptualizations can be dramatically affected by an ecological assessment. Two cases with the same *Diagnostic and Statistical Manual of Mental Disorders* (DSM) diagnosis would be seen differently, depending on the adolescents' life situations. For example, a 15-year-old girl may present to her family as having a conduct problem, but when assessed at school, teachers and peers find her to be a pleasant, academically engaged student. This case is radically different from that of a girl who is, for example, disruptive and truant in school but has positive relationships within her family. Both could conceivably fit the clinical diagnosis of conduct or oppositional defiant disorder. If a counselor has access to school information, the two cases can be differentiated readily. If the counselor is working within the school, the intervention options expand to a wider range within the ecological cube. For example, a weekly home–school communication system might be all that is needed to address the issues of the adolescent student whose difficulty seems limited to the school setting.

The best programs rely extensively on structured assessments for determining the target and form of interventions, including clinical work in schizophrenia (Paul & Menditto, 1992), child and family therapy (Sanders & Lawton, 1993), adult substance abuse (Miller & Rollnick, 2002), and marital therapy (Weiss, Halford, & Kim, 1996). In the multilevel model described in Chapter 4, decisions about the level of need and motivation to change are based on assessment.

ADDRESSING COMORBIDITY

The fourth feature of an ecological approach is the explicit effort to address the profile of adjustment problems (i.e., comorbidity) with adolescents and families in one comprehensive intervention strategy. For instance, does a 14-year-old girl who uses marijuana and alcohol, is arrested for shoplifting, and is depressed, get diagnosed and treated as having a conduct disorder or as an adolescent with major depression?

Children and families do not present themselves in neat diagnostic packages. To address the dynamics of real-world settings and people, we base interventions on an assessment of behavior across settings, as well as on current family dynamics. The linkage between assessment and intervention suggests that such interventions show "structured flexibility." In the example previously mentioned, the intervention response may depend on the scenario. The 14-year-old girl might be living in a recently reconstituted family, with a new stepfather and a new baby. Previously, the girl may have lived alone with her 39-year-old mother. Since the remarriage, her life may have changed dramatically. Compare this scenario with that of a girl whose family situation has been stable since birth, but who has been victimized at school because of some aspect of her appearance. Two divergent ecologies with similar symptom patterns suggest two different case conceptualizations, and quite possibly, intervention strategies. The difference in case conceptualizations may not be captured completely within a clinical interview with the parent or adolescent. We find that direct observation and assessments at home and at school often unveil dynamics that are unknown to the adolescent and family.

In this sense, we frequently find that careful assessment, accompanied by a flexible but empirically supported intervention menu,

provides an optimal framework for dealing with the clinical heterogeneity we see in real-world settings. As we discuss later, flexibility
and intervention menus are also critical to motivation and engagement. This applies to the content and process of an intervention. Interventions designed to build motivation provide a menu of change
strategies to optimize client engagement (Miller & Rollnick, 2002).
Direct interactions with clients that prioritize therapy process, rather
than the curriculum, facilitate behavior change as well (Patterson &
Chamberlain, 1994; Rogers, 1940).

At the onset, it may seem overwhelmingly complex to design an
intervention program within a ecological framework, but it is not. In
the next section, we describe our "tiered" approach to intervention
in ATP. We expect that the more comprehensive approach can be delivered by a full-time school counselor, with the appropriate training
to work collaboratively with parents and school professionals, and
with the appropriate resources, such as media and the support of
school staff.

THE MULTILEVEL ATP STRATEGY

A "Tiered" Intervention System

It is possible to address all levels of the ecological cube by systematically linking the levels, targets, and intervention methods within a
comprehensive, tiered strategy. In a "tiered" strategy, each level of intervention builds on the previous level. In traditional nomenclature,
the three levels represent universal (prevention), selected (at risk),
and indicated (treatment) family interventions. The universal level
reaches all youth and parents within a school setting; the selected
level addresses the needs of at-risk youth and families; and the indicated level is best described as adolescent and family treatment
(model displayed in Figure 2.2). We briefly provide an overview of
the three-tiered strategy of the ATP model. Later chapters describe
each level in more detail.

Universal Level

To implement a family-centered intervention within an existing service delivery system, considerable groundwork needs to take place
(1) to encourage appropriate referrals, to link the various services to-

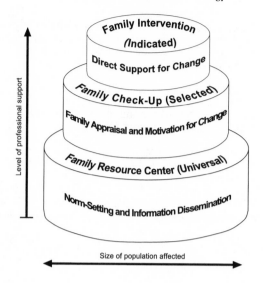

FIGURE 2.2. The multilevel ATP intervention strategy.

gether with a system, and to manage engagement; (2) to reach parents with information about services; (3) to disseminate parenting information; and (4) to educate and to consult and coordinate with professionals within schools and the community about accurate identification and empirically supported services to adolescents and families.

With a school system, the first step toward this goal is to establish a Family Resource Center (FRC). The FRC also provides the vehicle through which a program of multilevel interventions can be offered during the school year. For example, a public middle school hires a full-time professional to staff an FRC. She spends her day engaged in a variety of activities, including direct interventions with parents of high-risk students; consulting with teachers and principals on student intervention plans; attending health classes, with the goal of adding parent outreach components; monitoring individual students; and providing feedback to parents. Strategies used in conjunction with the FRC are described in detail in Chapter 9. Figure 2.3 summarizes the services provided through the FRC. This level of intervention is described as universal because it provides an infrastructure service that potentially affects all students, including those at low risk.

- School orientation meeting for parents (self-check, books, and videotapes, *Parenting in the Teenage Years*, by Dishion, Kavanagh, & Christianson, 1995)

- Media on effective parenting and norms

- Classroom-based parent–child exercises that support family management practices

- Communication of specific information to parents about attendance, behavior, and completion of assignments

- Screening and assessment

FIGURE 2.3. Universal intervention: Family Resource Center.

Risk Identification

A basic piece of the infrastructure of an FRC is to identify pro-actively students who are on a path leading to more serious adjustment problems. We used a gating strategy for this identification and for further parent engagement. The gating metaphor, adopted from earlier work on multistage screening for high-risk behavior, describes the successive assessment-based screening and resource allocation to families on the continuum of risk (Cronbach & Glesar, 1965; Dishion & Patterson, 1992; Loeber, Dishion, & Patterson, 1984; Walker & Severson, 1991).

There are a variety of ways to identify parents at the selected level for the FCU. In our work on the multiple-gating strategy, we used teacher ratings as the first assessment, followed by an assessment of family management as the second gate (Dishion & Patterson, 1992; Loeber & Dishion, 1987; Loeber et al., 1984). Our approach to family assessment is described in more detail in Chapter 3.

The development of a multiple-gating strategy is empirically justified but potentially harmful from a community psychology perspective. Like all assessment strategies, teacher ratings are highly predictive (see Loeber & Dishion, 1983), but also biased. We systematically examined the teacher ratings of problem behavior for sixth- and seventh-grade middle school students in a multiethnic urban setting.

Unfortunately, we found that teacher ratings of risk were highest for minority males, so to assess the validity of these ratings, we controlled for peer nominations, self-report, and school records of school behavior. Even after controlling for all three alternative sources on problem behavior, teacher ratings were still higher for minority males (Kavanagh, Burraston, Dishion, & Schneiger, 2000).

We suggest caution in using teachers' ratings to identify students proactively within a school setting that serves diverse students. Teacher identification of risk may be a poor first step in the process of engaging parents in parenting resources and promoting home–school collaboration. Consultation with and training for teachers to improve the validity of their judgments about risk, and to use constructive strategies for communicating to parents, is an important part of implementing the ATP in a school setting. In Chapter 9, we suggest implementation ideas for a gating strategy of risk assessment that is sensitive to the school and family context.

The Family Check-Up

Whether working in schools or in an outpatient clinic, adolescents and their families are referred because of specific concerns about their behavior in the home, school, or community.

The optimal condition for building parent motivation is self-identification. This typically occurs when parents come to the FRC because of concerns about their adolescents' adjustment at home or at school. A second motivation-enhancing opportunity occurs when parents are notified of discipline problems in the school. FRC staff should be part of school staffing committees, in order to catch problems early and make recommendations for family intervention, as opposed to child intervention, which is typical of schools.

Once FRC personnel become part of school staff, teachers, counselors, or administrators with concerns over behavior, peer associations, or emotional adjustment may refer a child proactively. To promote parental engagement, it is best to have school personnel recommend the FCU as a way to gather more information that would be important to both the family and the school in designing a plan to promote success and well-being during the teenage years.

The FCU was designed to handle the initial stage of a direct intervention with a family. As such, it is thought of as a selected intervention, because prior to an assessment, we only know that a youth and his family are at risk for problem behavior. As described in more detail in Chapter 5, the FCU is an in-depth method that supports parents' accurate appraisal of their child's risk status and provides parenting resources for reducing risk factors and promoting adjustment. The FCU, based on motivational interviewing by Miller and Rollnick (2002), is a three-session intervention: (1) the initial interview; (2) a comprehensive multiagent, multimethod assessment; and (3) a family feedback session that uses motivational skills to encourage maintenance of current positive practices and change of parenting problems. Feedback to parents based on a reliable, valid, and sensitive family assessment is a powerful tool for building parental motivation to engage in appropriate intervention resources (Sanders & Lawton, 1993).

The Family Intervention Menu

The indicated level of intervention provides direct professional support to parents to change clinically significant adjustment problems such as behavior, emotional well-being, and substance use. The presumption underlying the menu of family intervention services is that a variety of family-centered interventions can be equally effective in reducing problem behavior. Research by Weber (1998) unexpectedly revealed that the number of behavioral family therapy sessions was uncorrelated to clinically significant change. Perhaps Webster-Stratton most convincingly demonstrated that a variety of intervention formats is effective for families with problematic preschoolers (Webster-Stratton, 1984; Webster-Stratton et al., 1988).

The indicated intervention menu includes a brief family intervention, school monitoring system, parent groups, behavioral family therapy, and case management services. Given this model, our menu of intervention options is grounded in family management practices. However, as discussed in other areas of counseling and clinical psychology (Miller & Rollnick, 2002), it motivates the change process to have a variety of intervention options. The Family Management Curriculum (FMC; Dishion et al., 2003) provides a framework for working with families in groups (Chapter 6), with adolescents individually (Chapter 7), or with individual families (Chapter 8). The menu of intervention services potentially offered to parents, based on the FCU, is provided in Figure 2.4.

- Family Management Group

- Home–school card

- One-to-two sessions on special topics
  (Family Management Curriculum)

- Monthly monitoring

- Individual family management therapy
  (Family Management Curriculum)

- Referrals to more intensive services

FIGURE 2.4. Indicated intervention: support for family management.

An Outpatient Strategy

The preceding discussion is relevant to developing family-centered intervention within a community mental health clinic. The first gate, of course, is the family's self-identification that it needs services (i.e., making a telephone call, walking through the door of the clinic). As we all know, many adolescent referrals either come through the school or the juvenile court, so it is wise to link an outpatient service to the referral needs of a school district or juvenile justice system. Many outpatient services follow this strategy as a matter of course to survive economically, because most mental health services to children, adolescents, and families currently are not covered by mental health insurance. In these clinical situations, a school referral or an arrest serves as a clinically significant first gate in the service delivery system.

We understand that many readers will be working outside of a school, or other service delivery system, with families who may be considered at risk or high risk (selected or indicated). Much of the focus of this book is on our direct-service model, summarized in Figure 2.5, which has two broad phases. The first, *engagement and motivation*, is the topic of Chapters 3, 4, and 5. The second, *implementation of a family intervention menu*, includes Chapters 6, 7, and 8. Finally, in Chapters 9, 10, and 11, we address broader issues related to implementing the intervention in service settings and evaluating impact as a foundation for change.

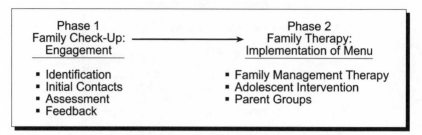

FIGURE 2.5. Two phases of the ATP intervention model.

SUMMARY

This chapter has provided an overview of the ATP multilevel strategy. The ecological cube was introduced and discussed as the foundation for the design of the ATP intervention model. Consistent with our family-centered model, our intervention program is concerned with engagement of parents and support of family management.

We now proceed to discuss, in more detail, the basic issues of engagement and motivation when working with families of adolescents.

PART II

The Family Check-Up
Engaging and Motivating Family Change

Although it is clear that family-centered interventions are empirically effective (Kazdin, 2002; Taylor & Biglan, 1998), it is less than obvious how to engage parents to the level that would impact the community (Spoth, Kavanagh, & Dishion, 2002). It is often difficult to recruit parents to participate in parent groups or family therapy, and when they do participate, they often drop out before completing a protocol. The engagement issues are especially challenging for parents of adolescents (Dishion & Patterson, 1992).

Following our experiences of applying family-centered interventions to unselected, community samples, we became convinced that the literature on the effectiveness of family-centered interventions underestimates the engagement problem. As suggested above, this may be due to the role of research funding in engaging families to participate in intervention studies. Even though parents are often not paid for interventions (with notable exceptions; see Fleischman, 1979), payment for assessments associated with the intervention is often quite high. In addition, well-funded research staff are able to find study participants (Capaldi, Chamberlain, Fetrow, & Wilson, 1997).

Miller and Rollnick (2002) designed a set of techniques, referred to as *motivational interviewing*, that addresses the problem of engagement and motivation. These procedures actually emerged from the therapy process literature on parent resistance to behavioral family therapy (e.g., Patterson & Chamberlain, 1994; Patterson & Forgatch, 1985), and the stages-of-change model in treatment for addictions (Prochaska & DiClemente, 1986; Prochaska, Velicer, Guadagnoli, & Rossi, 1991). There is also a strong connection between motivational interviewing and a client-centered approach to counseling, articulated by Carl Rogers (1940) over 60 years ago.

Motivational interviewing addresses the client's stage of change before engaging in interventions design to enact change. Miller and colleagues developed the Drinker's Check-Up based on these procedures (Miller & Rollnick, 2002). This brief, motivational intervention was found to be as effective as 28 days of inpatient treatment for effecting long-term reductions in problem drinking (Miller & Sovereign, 1989). One of the key strategies for building motivation to change in addiction is to provide a "menu" of intervention options. For example, although clients involved in the Drinker's Check-Up did not initially agree to residential treatment, many sought such support to change their drinking practices after attempting to control their problem drinking on their own (Brown & Miller, 1993). It is motivating for clients to be able to take their first step in the change process based on their preference for a list of available resources. Also noteworthy is that over 90% of the unselected community samples that quit smoking did so on their own, without the help of a professional. Although there are many differences when comparing smoking cessation with family change, we think the same principle applies to family-centered intervention.

Motivational interviewing inspired our work on engaging and motivating parents, and our design of the Family Check-Up. The Family Check-Up is a three-session intervention that includes an initial contact, an assessment session, and a feedback interview. Chapters 3, 4, and 5 describe each of these phases of the Family Check-Up in detail.

3

Initial Strategies for Family Engagement

In this chapter, we discuss strategies for establishing a collaborative helping relationship with families, and how to avoid common pitfalls in the initial stages of work with a family. We also discuss strategies for building a positive foundation for change (such as establishing a comprehensive assessment), a family-relationship perspective, and motivating family engagement.

An initial contact can occur in a variety of settings and circumstances. For example, contacts can occur in the family's home, in a school principal's office, in the juvenile court, in a mental health clinic, or more commonly, on the telephone. Our experience is that families can be turned off to the change process by initial interactions that unintentionally foreclose self-appraisal, motivation, confidence in services, and ultimately, the change process.

CLINICAL LOGISTICS

In many situations, initial interactions occur with parents via telephone. These seemingly trivial contacts are actually a critical step in establishing the collaborative relationship. Caregivers can begin from a place of blaming the teenager ("He is hyperactive, traumatized, depressed, bipolar, attention deficit," and so forth) or others (e.g., spouse, ex-spouse) for the problem. The stories and blame are part and parcel of experiences of interpersonal distress, but carry many traps that can serve as barriers to effective engagement. Structure the initial contacts to be friendly, respectful, and optimistic, but concrete with respect to the concerns of the parent, the urgency and risk of the situation, and scheduling the first meeting.

The function of the initial contact is to understand the family situation with respect to engagement in a family-centered service. In the first intake call, it is important to identify the adults who serve in a caregiving role, sibling issues, family member schedules, and family members' willingness to participate. Questions and discussions should focus specifically on family members' involvement: "Would Bill be interested in talking with us about this issue?"

Caregivers may not understand the need to bring in partners or other family members (e.g., a grandmother or aunt). Until recently, parents often were confused by their own involvement in therapy. It may be helpful to structure questions that help broaden the issue to include other caregivers:

> "From what you've said, it sounds like a good time to take some action. Who else in your family shares your concern about this situation?"

The telephone contact is the initial step in the change process. As such, we may engage unwittingly or collude with an existing dynamic that may potentially undermine change. A mother who excludes a father because of his work schedule inadvertently may be fulfilling a script in which she alone is responsible for parenting issues. The father's lack of engagement could also be a major part of the problem—his work becomes a convenient excuse to disengage from his marriage and family. On the other hand, the mother's involvement in therapy without her partner may be the first step in extricating herself and her children from an abusive relationship.

The initial contact is not meant to determine which of these scenarios apply. Extended discussions of the parents' story about the problem should be deferred to an intake interview. The focus is to represent accurately the family-centered approach to service delivery and to respect the parents' initial judgments about how the collaboration should start. Also, assume that the constellation of participants will change over time. For example, a family with joint custody may eventually involve the second parent, because the child-rearing routines of two houses usually require coordination and discussion to address the behavior of an adolescent. We have worked with all combinations of family members, including, at times, just the adolescent (see Chapter 7).

If appropriate, an intake is scheduled and a Family Intake Questionnaire—Adolescent Version (FIQ-A), map, and parking information are sent to families. Ideally, the initial contact meeting is scheduled for about 90 minutes, to provide enough time for an overview of the services of the clinic, to address confidentiality, to review informed consent, to complete an intake form, and to conduct the initial contact. This is the ideal world of an outpatient clinic, and families that are appointment-oriented can read and complete an intake form independently. These are also families whose adolescents and parenting partners are cooperative and agree to meeting with a therapist.

The FIQ-A provides preliminary information about marital status, household constitution and caregiving structure, problem behavior in the "target child" and siblings, developmental issues, friendships, stress level, family strengths, past trauma and present contextual disrupters, use of mental health services, and positive activities.

The FIQ-A also provides a summary of the results of the intake and gives an excellent form from which to develop the preliminary case conceptualization. It is especially important to have caregivers evaluate which of the behaviors on the questionnaire are a "problem" for the parent, and for which they would like help. Chamberlain and Reid (1987) found that such targeted problem behaviors are most likely to change when using the Parent Daily Report (PDR) as a measure of clinical outcome.

Commonly, parents lose or forget to complete the FIQ-A prior to the intake interview. If time allows, having them complete the questionnaire immediately prior to the meeting will help alleviate this possibility. Allow parents an opportunity to look over their answers and to make notes about issues requiring clarification, or that you wish to discuss further.

INITIAL INTERVIEW

We prefer to conduct the initial interview as a semistructured interview. The FIQ-A allows the therapist to focus on key areas of concern that are relevant to the family's current situation and the ensuing engagement in the change process. For example, a history of domestic violence raises unique clinical concerns that should be addressed initially when working with a parent. As the therapist, be aware of restraining orders and other procedures developed to protect a child or parent from future violence or abuse. The therapist is in a better position to establish a solid collaboration with a parent if issues such as these can be addressed in the initial contacts. Hearing about a history of child abuse when walking out the door at the end of an initial interview suggests to all participants that a solid collaborative relationship has yet to be established.

We discourage reviewing the FIQ-A in detail in the company of parents or adolescents. Too much attention to a form or questionnaire when meeting with a parent or adolescent disrupts the process of listening and focusing on reflecting and understanding their perspective vis-à-vis motivation to change and the family relationship perspective (Miller & Rollnick, 2002).

The therapist typically begins with initial questions that can structure the course of the discussion, for example, "Tell me in your own words about your concerns for Lupé and your family." To get more detail about a possible safety issue, an opening question such as the following might apply: "I see that you had a restraining order on your ex-husband. How is that situation now?" Questions such as this provide direction and structure, but allow the parent to bring the therapist into the present circumstance of her life.

Ideally, we have two therapists meet with the adolescent and parent simultaneously. In this way, we meet with the family together to discuss the logistics of the intake interview, then separate for about 40 minutes. Optimally, the family reconvenes at the end of the initial contact, with the parent's therapist summarizing the parent's decision about the next step. At that time, the adolescent's therapist may wish to summarize the adolescent's interests in the family change process.

The priority from a family-centered perspective is to meet with the parent. If there is only one therapist, meet with the parent first, then with the adolescent. Alternatively, schedule a first meeting with the parent and a second with the adolescent and parent together. Discussions of the adolescent's problem behavior, divorced partners, and so forth, must be minimized in the presence of the adolescent. Families often terminate the therapy because the adolescent refuses to attend. This emphasizes the importance of establishing a strong collaborative relationship with the parent initially, in order to reduce the vulnerability to dropout as a result of the teenager's resistance to change.

Differences in level of concern, availability, trust in mental health services, family dynamics, and other factors may limit the adults who participate in the initial interview. Flexibility to adjust and reconsider the original formulation of the family is critical at times. Consider the following example, and see how the definition of the family changed over time, during the course of the initial contacts:

> Dennis is a single father with two boys, both diagnosed with Asperger's syndrome; he is unemployed but receives disability.
> Dennis is overwhelmed with parenting and managing the demands of various social service agencies. Based on the telephone report and initial interview, it became clear that that his boys are in need of daily structure and a routine that helps them get to school on time and complete their homework.

These boys, although difficult to manage in the family home, were not drug-involved or delinquent. The diagnostic label of Asperger's, although not technically accurate, mobilized intervention resources for the family. On the other hand, the Asperger's label also distracted professionals from the functional dynamics driving the problem behavior. Despite all the services, the boys were falling rapidly behind in basic academic survival skills.

Over the telephone, and in the initial interview, it would have been easy to fall into the same pattern as other helping professionals. Despite his good intentions, Dennis did not communicate clearly and was unable to implement a parenting plan. The natural tendency for some therapists is to set up a system in which the father's role is less central. Unfortunately, this "therapeutic trap" never works in the long run, because chronically overloaded social service helpers, volunteers, and others who help with household routines always move on with their lives, leaving the family even less able to manage their children and their lives.

Fortunately, this family's therapist took a broader view of the family and actively solicited more information about the absent mother. She periodically became depressed and, during these episodes, often left the household. She returned when the depression subsided. During her 2- to 3-month absences, it was not unusual for the father to seek help from low-cost services in the community.

After the therapist talked with the mother and father separately, the family agreed to participate in the family assessment as a unit. The assessment revealed hidden strengths that would not have been seen otherwise. We gradually worked on improving the partnership of the mother and father, and eventually the family was reconstituted. Our work with family members focused on supporting better strategies for coping with the dynamics of their lives, as well as making better use of the services available to the family. This case illustrates the importance of exploring assumptions and options at the initial stages of contact. Also, in this case, proper attention to the absentee mother as a resource empowered a reorganization within the family and an adjustment of the services previously experienced as ineffective.

INITIAL ENGAGEMENT STRATEGIES

Channeling

In the initial contact, the therapist's work is to channel individual points of view into a family-relationship perspective. This is a neutral statement of the family's current situation that is acceptable and conducive to change for the entire family. A classic example is that of the teenager who wants more freedom and the parent who is upset by problem behaviors such as substance use, partying with friends, and poor schoolwork. The difference in perspectives leads to a cycle of conflict, coercion, and perhaps, eventually, the adolescent's breaking of family ties.

The family perspective promotes family relationships as a priority. It provides a shift from the content of the problem, to the process of interacting as a family. A family-relationship perspective might be the following:

"Okay, from everything I've heard from you and Ramon, it would be helpful for your family to find a way to talk about and agree on the expectations for Ramon for the rest of the school year. Let's find a way for you to deal with this issue without fighting."

This statement serves no guarantee of the full collaboration of all family members, but it does provide an opportunity to move the discussion forward and potentially build motivation to have an assessment and feedback session. The family relationship perspective is the first step in turning the problem into a solution, as shown in Figure 3.1. In this way, the past, present, and future are linked by a pragmatic goal: Where does the family go from here?

Note that the ultimate goal is to understand every family member's perspective in order to ensure equity, fairness, and compassion for *all* family members. Realistically, initial contacts may be limited to only one or two individuals within the family. However, to channel the perspective of family members into a family-relationship perspective, it is necessary to engage clinically both the parent *and* the adolescent. Below, we discuss strategies to facilitate interactions we have found to be useful for engagement.

Parental Engagement

The initial interview with the parent should rely on basic strategies in motivational interviewing (Miller & Rollnick, 2002), with respect to understanding the parent's motivational space. Consistent with Prochaska and DiClemente's (1982, 1986) empirically based conceptualization, we might think of family members in the precontemplation or contemplation stage at the intake interview. Rarely do we interact with a parent who is ready to take action, or who is in

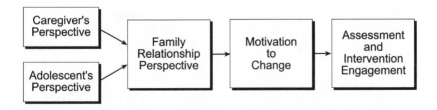

FIGURE 3.1. Channeling diverse perspectives into positive family change.

the maintenance-of-change stage. If families are in crisis, however, they may well be in the action stage, but only relative to handling the crisis. They may not see how the patterns of family mismanagement and disruption place them in a state of crisis. To work within their understanding of the dynamics leading to crises, it is often important to handle the crisis first. Consider the following situation:

> Ebony was a 21-year-old trapped in a 14-year-old's body. She and her older sister (age 16, no longer attending high school) spent most of their free time at the apartment of a group of young men known for partying and some drug sales. Ebony's European American father and African American mother had no influence on her. If they set limits on Ebony, she left and did not return for 3 or 4 days.
>
> A Family Check-Up was out of the question until the family stabilized. The therapist worked only with the parents (Ebony would not attend an intake session) to develop plans for Ebony for the summer. When she returned, the parents and Ebony were more closely aligned, and a Family Check-Up and family therapy were pursued.

When families are in crisis, support is needed to manage the turmoil before long-term support for change can be provided. Empirically successful approaches to working with families of adolescents demonstrate that in working with highly disorganized, chaotic families, home visits and crisis management are the best means for improving family functioning and reducing adolescent problem behavior (Henggeler et al., 1998).

Statistically, the more prevalent clinical scenario is that at least one parent is in the contemplation stage in the behavior-change cycle. Figure 3.2 summarizes some basic interviewing strategies that specifically address the emotional issues of seeking help for parenting. These strategies are seen as complementing the motivational interviewing that accompanies any initial clinical contact.

1. *Support effort.* Parenting can be a black box. If you are not successful, it looks and feels like you have done nothing. It is absolutely essential that we find and support parenting efforts. Parents need to know that you understand they have been trying. At a very minimum, the fact that they show up for an intake interview and complete a questionnaire requires effort and courage:

✓ Support effort.

✓ Paraphrase and clarify efforts.

✓ Reflect discrepancies.

✓ Link concerns with services.

✓ Create optimistic reframes.

FIGURE 3.2. Strategies for parent engagement.

"It's clear to me that even though you're getting upset with Ebony, the fact that you're here shows you're doing everything you can to keep her safe and in the family."

2. *Paraphrase and clarify concerns.* Again, understanding the parent's primary concern is the basic work of the intake interview. Parents will respond to a therapist who works to understand; this process can go a long way toward repairing any mistakes or breaches in the emerging therapeutic relationship:

"Oh, I'm sorry. I see what you're saying. It's not that you want to change John's personality. You're worried that if he's this impulsive now, when it comes time to drive, he'll do something crazy and hurt himself or someone else."

3. *Reflect discrepancies.* This is a central strategy of motivational interviewing. When talking to parents, it is common to hear conflicting and competing emotions. These discrepancies are the grist of the motivational mill. Listen carefully and reflect these discrepancies during the initial interview. In this way, the therapist can scaffold the parent's process of working through what is the most important first step for family change.

"It seems like it's a little unclear to you whether your problems with Ebony are disrupting your marriage or if your disagreements about parenting are creating the problems."

4. *Link concerns to assessment.* By the end of the initial contact, it is critical that there be a clear sense of how the services you offer genuinely address the parents' concerns. At the end of the initial contact, if it seems appropriate for an assessment of the family's interaction process or the child's school behavior, it will be evident and obvious to both the parents and the therapist.

> "Given what we said, it might be helpful to take a close look at how the family communicates and deals with conflict, so you can get a handle on what to do now."

5. *Co-create an optimistic understanding.* Turning an adolescent's problem behavior into a positive prognostic sign is a useful way to engage both parents and adolescents in the change process (Robins, Alexander, Newell, & Turner, 1996). This is a high-level therapeutic skill that needs practice and sensitivity. Given the complexity of family behavior, however, it is likely that even nasty behavior has "unintended" positive implications for family change.

> "I've seen this before in other stepparent families. Even though John seems to be negative with you (e.g., the stepparent), he also does a lot to keep you engaged in his life. Some teenagers wouldn't tell you so much—they would be sneaky."

A common strategy for supporting parents is to normalize their struggles and concerns. This is an excellent way of providing support, because there is no greater relief than to know that others in the world often share the same issues and struggles. However, normalizing does not always build engagement and motivation to change and, therefore, should be used mindfully.

> "You know, a lot of parents experience more conflict with their kids in adolescence. In this sense, your experiences aren't unusual, but the swearing and pushing between mom and daughter is a clear sign that things are getting out of control in your family."

It is noteworthy that by the teenage years, many families will have sought help previously and experienced some successes and failures (or perhaps treatment traumas). These past treatment experiences will undoubtedly have baggage, with respect to the family's engagement in services, openness to self-appraisal, and the change process. About half of young adolescents with arrest histories have been involved in some form of mental health treatment (Stouthamer-Loeber et al., 1995). When including school professionals, the percentage is likely much higher. The therapist must address previous professional experiences with special attention to individual family members' current motivational stance. These experiences, if left unattended, can serve as disruptive ghosts in the change process. If discussed, these experiences can form a basis for better understanding and perhaps a way to join with parents about those bad experiences. We discuss this issue when addressing issues of working with families during the change process.

Adolescent Engagement

Some therapists assume that to engage an adolescent, it is necessary to act like one; however, adolescents are acutely sensitive to adult attempts to "be liked" and presentations of a "false self." Be yourself and work hard to understand the uniqueness of this young adult's personality, strengths, and perspective on the family. It is impossible to generalize a set of concerns or interests of an adolescent, but there are some unique features of their developmental status in the family and community that can be addressed to promote engagement:

1. *Respect space and privacy.* Give a young person plenty of room to cooperate with the initial contact process and to discuss sensitive issues related to the family. The adolescent is often distrustful of mental health professionals and the therapy process, making it imperative that your initial gestures and interactions communicate respect for privacy. Plan ahead what the adolescent can do if he decides not to participate. Communicate that the pressure is off.

> "Okay, fair enough. Sounds like you weren't too happy about coming here today, and you aren't sure if you even want to talk to me."

2. *Normalize experiences.* This may be an important tool for working with adolescents, who are often concerned with being "normal." By virtue of a story about other adolescents you've worked

with, you can get to a place that opens doors for talking about feelings and experiences.

> "I know of a lot of young people who aren't always happy when their parents marry, even though everyone else seems to think it should be a happy occasion. Can you see feeling like that?"

This statement provides a possible bridge to having a frank discussion about an adolescent's obviously negative reaction to a recent stepparent marriage. If the teen says either "That makes no sense" or "That makes a lot of sense," it opens doors for further discussion.

3. *Advocate the adolescent's interests.* Early on, it is important to articulate the nature of your relationship with an adolescent client. You, as an adult, are going to use all your knowledge and skills to help this adolescent get along in a world of adults. For the teen, this may mean having fewer negative experiences at school, reducing the fighting at home with parents, improving the fairness of household rules, or keeping out of harm's way.

> "It sounds like things get out of control in your house when you and your parents disagree. One way we might work together is to figure out ways you can ask for things without the situation always turning into a fight."

Be careful not to oversell your advocacy and inadvertently collude with an adolescent to engage in behavior that puts her at risk on a variety of dimensions:

> "I see why you want to be with your boyfriend all the time. On the other hand, I know that any parent who gives a damn about their kids is going to have problems with that. Can you see your mom's point of view at all? What are some of the things she might worry about?"

Here, we understand the adolescent's reference point but are not selling out the parents' perspective or unintentionally colluding or supporting the view that the concerns of the adolescent's parents are inappropriate. To do so can further alienate young people from their delicately perilous protective shield of a family.

4. *Link interests with services.* Just like the parents, adolescents need to see the connection between their concerns, and the assessment and intervention that follows:

> "One of the services we provide is looking carefully at how family members communicate. We then use that information to help them get along better. It seems that most of us don't always understand why we act the way we do in family life, and it helps to have someone else look more closely."

5. *Create optimistic reframes.* Young people come to therapy with the idea that they are the problem, and that the therapy is really about fixing them. The implication is that their behavior is hurting the family. This implicit understanding feels bad and is not conducive to their discussing family issues, because the expectation is that all roads lead to Rome (meaning, their bad behavior). Robins et al. (1996) actually found that the effect of positive reframes on the adolescent's behavior was most strongly related to the adolescent's engagement in therapy:

> "This may sound funny, but I'm starting to see that you might be helping your parents out by distracting them from other worries. You might not even see this.
>
> "I can see that you and your dad fight a lot about chores. On the other hand, I'm impressed with your work skills, especially when you work for other people. Maybe it's the arguments that interfere with you helping more around the house."

6. *Keep it brief, start slow.* Many therapists err on the side of being too friendly, too intrusive, or both, with adolescents, which may be one of the major factors leading to adolescents resisting involvement in family therapy. Give them opportunities to disengage, and keep the intake session brief, unless otherwise indicated. One rule of thumb is a maximum of 30 minutes per session until adolescents are age 15 or 16.

> "Okay, we're not going to meet very long. I just want to make sure I get a chance to hear your point of view, so I can understand what you would like to see happen in the family."

The basic idea behind engaging adolescents in intervention services that adults believe are in the adolescents' best interests is much like the old proverb: "You can lead a horse to water but you can't force it to drink." To engage adolescents, you need to respect and label their initial posture in therapy, but continue to look for opportunities to support their motivation to improve their family situation. Respecting the parents' leadership role while also advocating the interests of the adolescent provides a solid foundation for eventual engagement. Be sensitive to the implied dynamics of the therapeutic situation. It may be difficult to establish a therapeutic alliance with an adolescent when the situation is loaded (e.g., a mother who brings an adolescent to discuss her recent marriage to a young male, if the therapist is a young male, may encounter some initial resistance).

The Next Step

As shown in Figure 3.3, it is necessary to engage key family participants to build a family relationship perspective that works for all involved. Once this is established, it is important to sell the family on the need for assessment before moving forward on their own, or with the help of professional services. Most families (and professionals) do not see the value of sound psychological assessment to their personal lives.

If we have the opportunity to meet with the adolescent and parents, we spend a brief time together as a group before the end of the

❶ Respect privacy and space.

❷ Normalize experiences.

❸ Advocate interests.

❹ Link interests with services.

❺ Create optimistic reframes.

❻ Keep it brief.

FIGURE 3.3. Strategies for adolescent engagement.

initial contact, then take the lead in summarizing what has been learned and the recommended next step. Some statements promote the family's investment in the assessment and feedback sessions:

> "From our talk today, it seems like the family agrees that the conflict has gotten out of control, especially around Ebony's time away from home and her school situation. I share the concern that in the long run, the situation is really going to hurt Ebony.
>
> "What I would recommend is that the family participate in the Family Check-Up. This involves two more meetings, the first of which is a careful assessment of how Ebony and the family are doing. It gives us a chance to see how things unfold in your home. We also assess how Ebony is doing at school in a variety of situations.
>
> "Then we study all this information and sit down with all of you and give you feedback. Many families really never have an opportunity to take a careful look at their situation before making critical life decisions. We offer you that service, and we'll also help you make sense of it in our feedback meetings.
>
> "Does this sound like it will be a useful service for you?"

It is important to leave enough time to discuss concerns or questions about the assessment and feedback sessions that follow. Most families, by this stage of the process, are willing to be involved in the assessment. Part of the reason for this motivational stance is that the therapist will point out to the parents, especially, how they may benefit from getting more information on an issue:

> "It would be helpful to you to have more detail on how Ebony gets along with other students at school, or You might want to take a closer look at how you work together to handle Ebony when she becomes challenging. That's why we always have a videotape family assessment task before we start working with a family."

This process of linking the family's concerns with the assessment services to follow, by and large, is an easy sell to parents and adolescents that more information can be helpful for solving a problem they are experiencing.

SUMMARY

In this chapter, we have discussed a variety of strategies to use in the initial contacts with a family. These contacts set the stage for a family's potential to change as they work with you, or in the future, if they see other helping professionals.

The task of the initial contacts is to form a bridge from a past problem to a future solution. Exploring parent and adolescent family appraisals, and finding a frame of reference that prioritizes improving the family management and communication processes, accomplishes this. The frame of reference should sell the family on how a careful assessment could help to determine the next step. Ideally, both parents and teenagers will be curious and interested in getting feedback on the family assessment.

We now turn to the rationale and procedures for conducting a comprehensive family assessment.

4

An Ecological Assessment Strategy

By ecological assessment, we refer to a broad assessment that includes the youth's behavior and emotional adjustment, academic behavior, peer relations, contextual influences on the family, and family interaction patterns. The inclusion of a structured ecological assessment, prior to engagement of the family into intervention services, is an indispensable and unique feature of the ATP and the ecological approach, in general (Dishion & Stormshak, in press). We use assessments to improve collaborative decision making between the therapist and family, and as a key strategy for building motivation to change. This chapter provides the details needed to conduct our basic assessment, or for use in adapting an assessment that better fits intervention and service delivery needs.

A BRIEF RATIONALE

Interventions with adolescents and families require complex decision making and judgment. For example, therapists often make decisions about how frequently to meet, which intervention targets to prioritize (parenting, adolescent's anger, parenting practices, mother's depression), and the frequency and intensity of the intervention (weekly, monthly, biweekly, daily). Theoretical perspectives often help simplify the decision-making task but do not seem to improve the overall quality of the outcome.

In most family-centered approaches, there are two solutions to this complex problem. The first is to provide an intervention program for parenting in which "one size fits all." This usually involves a parent group with a curriculum (see Dishion & Andrews, 1995; Dishion et al., 2003). The other approach is for the therapist, based on her clinical judgment, to make a series of decisions about the "best way" to work with a family or parent.

The problem with the former approach, as discussed earlier, is that having only one venue within which to work with families may be demotivating, thereby limiting the potential public health impact. The problem with the second approach, which depends on the therapist's judgment and decisions, is that (1) parents are often in a one-down position with the therapist from the beginning, and (2) clinical judgments have serious limitations when it comes to case conceptualization. In fact, the best way to improve clinical judgment is for therapists to use structured assessments and base decisions on data (Dawes, 1994).

We have known for some time that clinical decision making can be substantially improved by the use of psychological assessments (Dawes & Corrigan, 1974; Duncan, Ohlin, Reiss, & Stanton, 1953; Meehl & Rosen, 1955). In addition, we know that sharing assessment results with families can enhance their engagement and their own potential for making meaningful decisions about their family (Sanders & Lawton, 1993). The use of a structured approach to conduct assessments is what differentiates the ecological approach to clinical and counseling psychology from an eclectic approach: Assessments drive the use of a variety of empirically supported interventions.

THE MEASUREMENT STRATEGY

A Standard Battery

Clinical assessment too often focuses on identifying client deficits. The goal of an ecological assessment is to provide an overview of adolescent and family adjustment across the domains specified in our family-centered model (see Figure 1.1). These include the adolescent's adjustment, family context, family management, peer relationships, academic competence, and strengths and weaknesses, which are the foundation of both motivational interviewing and case conceptualization in a strength-based approach to intervention.

An important foundation is the assessment of family interaction. To better understand family dynamics and management practices, we conduct videotaped assessments in the home. Many professionals respond to this aspect of our assessment as too intrusive and costly for their own setting. We argue, however, that the assessment of family interaction is critical for motivating change. Because family interaction patterns are rarely cognitively accessible to participants (Patterson et al., 1992), it is often necessary to provide videotape feedback. Therefore, the omission of direct observation potentially undermines the ability of the therapist to facilitate the parents' shift in the appraisal that is necessary for building motivating change in family relationships.

To fully understand the relationship dynamics relevant to adolescent problem behavior, it would be ideal to assess both peer and family interactions directly. From a family-centered intervention model, however, it is more likely that changes in the peer group will be guided and maintained by parents (Dishion, Bullock, & Granic, 2002). Therefore, we prioritize the assessment of family interactions up to middle adolescence. It is interesting that videotaping of family interaction in the home is often experienced by families of different socioeconomic backgrounds as interesting and relevant to their family concerns.

A second critical feature of our assessment is to collect data from multiple reporting sources to compare *perceptions* of strengths and weaknesses. Kellam (1990) makes the important point that perceptions and objective measures of interaction provide two unique vantage points relevant to the youngster and family's situation and conceptualization. Combining the reports of significant others to create composite scores can mask variation that is critical to case conceptualization. For example, if teachers perceive a child to be problematic, but the parent or child himself does not, that is an important, clinically relevant variation. Achenbach (1992) addresses this issue in the scoring and conceptualization of the Child Behavior Checklist (CBCL) data of child adjustment across settings. Multiple reporting sources afford the opportunity to compare perceptions of teachers, mother, and father separately, and the youth, in the family feedback sessions.

Sampling the Ecology

We conceptualize the measurement and feedback in terms of risk and protective factors within each of three domains: child adjustment, peer adjustment, and family management and contextual influences (information on the standard assessment battery of measures we developed is available on the Child and Family Center website, *http:// cfc.uoregon.edu*). Consistent with an ecological approach to assessment, we include macroratings from significant others, direct observations of targeted family management practices, and structured reports to assess change in adolescent behavior over time (Dishion & Stormshak, in press).

The complete assessment requires approximately 2 hours, from initial interview through the interaction task and the additional time it takes the family to complete questionnaires between meetings. We make every effort to keep the standard assessment battery relatively brief. If clinical issues are raised in the intake interview (e.g., trauma), we may add other assessment procedures to focus on this specific issue. All family members are informed that summaries of their reports (not specific items) will be used for the purpose of making decisions in the best interest of the child and family, emphasizing that honest reporting is to everyone's advantage.

ASSESSMENT PROCEDURES

Questionnaires

If there is consensus between the parent and therapist for a Family Check-Up (FCU), the appropriate consent forms for release of information are signed, and the family is sent home with separate questionnaire packets for both the parent(s) and the child. Before leaving, arrangements are made to complete the Family Assessment Task (FAsTask), either in the family home, in the Family Resource Center (FRC), or in some other designated confidential meeting place. When scheduling the assessment, parents should be told that questionnaires must be completed by the next meeting, so that all the information can be compiled for the feedback meeting. If there are reading problems, family chaos, or concerns about family members sharing information, it is best to schedule separate times to complete the questionnaires, followed by another appointment for the FAsTask.

School Data

Regardless of a parent's perceptions of her youth's adjustment at school, it is essential to have at least one teacher complete ratings on social, academic, and emotional adjustment. Again, with a strength-based assessment strategy, positive peer relations or academic competence in the youth, despite problem behavior at home, is extremely important to case conceptualization and, consequently, the formulation of an intervention menu. Additionally, comparison of teacher, parent, and youth reports gives a sense of variation in behavior, perceptual biases, or both (Dishion & Stormshak, in press).

Teachers of middle school students often underestimate their sense of a child's peer relations, because they work with students for as little as 1 hour a day, typically under limited circumstances for social interaction. However, even under such circumstances, many teachers have a sense of a student's social standing and provide accurate predictions about long-term outcomes for students (see Loeber & Dishion, 1983). We seek out the teacher who is most likely to have a sense of a student's adjustment and, at times, supplement the assessment with a brief interview or teacher ratings to get not only a comprehensive picture of the resources for a specific student within a school setting but also the student's "pattern" of school adjustment.

Family Interactions

The videotaped FAsTask is a direct observation measure of family management practices: relationship quality, encouragement (positive reinforcement), limit setting, monitoring, problem solving, and norm setting. We derive a coercive process index (CPI) and a positive process index (PPI) from the videotaped interactions. Scores for these constructs are derived from a family management macrorating measure that can be completed by research assistants or therapists working with families. The use of structured, videotaped interactions to assess close relationships builds on the vast literature of family and marital interaction assessment (e.g., Forgatch, Fetrow, & Lathrop, 1985; Gottman, 1979; Weiss et al., 1996).

Direct observation is more appropriate for families from a wide range of socioeconomic and cultural backgrounds. Parents who did not finish high school, for example, are less amenable to completing wordy questionnaires and lengthy interviews designed by researchers with advanced graduate degrees. Videotaped interactions of family functioning are becoming a more common component in the assessment of diverse populations (Chase-Lansdale, Brooks-Gunn, & Zamsky, 1994; Gorman-Smith & Tolan, 1998). Interactional assessments, in fact, render intervention services that are beneficial for a broader cultural range of families. Again, the issue is complex, especially when the observer has a different ethnic background than that of the person being observed. In clinical assessment, however, we have known for some time that it is more difficult for a family in distress to "fake good" than for a nondistressed family to "fake bad" (Bolstad & Johnson, 1972). The more distressed the family (low false–negative error rate), the more useful direct observations of family interaction become.

The FAsTask takes about 1 hour to complete. For approximately half the observation session, the target child and parent (or parents) are videotaped in discussion. The remainder of the task includes the entire family (the task is appropriate for children 11 years and older) and involves a series of structured discussions that attempt to elicit interaction patterns relevant to family management. The FAsTask is broken down into structured interactions:

1. *5 minutes:* Parents and child plan an activity (relationship quality).
2. *5 minutes:* Parents lead a discussion about a positive child behavior they wish to encourage (encouraging growth).
3. *5 minutes:* Youth leads a discussion about a time he was without adult supervision (monitoring).
4. *5 minutes:* Parents lead a discussion of setting limits over the previous month (limit setting).
   [*Take a 5-minute break, after which all family members are brought in.*]
5. *5 minutes:* Entire family discusses a family problem that parents have preselected (problem solving).
6. *7 minutes:* Parents lead a discussion on the family beliefs about tobacco, alcohol, marijuana, or other substance use (drug-use norms).
7. *7 minutes:* Family plans a celebration together—not a birthday or regularly scheduled holiday (relationship quality).

The FAsTask ends with a 3-minute opportunity to give positive recognition to the child, allowing the task to end on a positive note. The therapist providing the family feedback should review the video-tape with care and complete the macroratings on family management and process. In this way, the therapist bases case conceptualization on carefully considered patterns of family interaction. In addition, videotape feedback is an effective way to motivate change and rein-force strengths.

Children and families do not always present themselves in neat packages, so it may be necessary to design a task that is more rele-vant to the clinical problem of interest. For example, when an eating disorder is suspected, the limit-setting task might be changed to dis-cuss family dietary practices. Although norms are not available for these variations, the approach the family takes to discussing relevant clinical issues is invaluable for working collaboratively to support change.

Intervention Process Measures

We also provide a tool for assessment of child adjustment that is sensitive to change. Building on the work of Chamberlain and Reid (1987), we use the PDR and the CDR. These assessments provide inexpensive measurement tools for assessing immediate family re-actions to intervention efforts, which involve periodic, brief tele-phone interviews with parent(s) and youth on symptoms and fam-ily events.

The clinical uses of a daily parent report were originally formu-lated and discussed by Patterson, Reid, Jones, and Conger (1975). We developed Parent Daily Report (PDR) and Child Daily Report (CDR) forms that are appropriate for adolescents age 11 and older. The major issue with daily reports is the repeated-measures effect. Regardless of the reporting agent, the first telephone call results in higher rates of reported problems (Chamberlain & Reid, 1987), so we suggest eliminating the first call from the summary score. Cham-berlain and Reid also found that three calls provide a stable estimate for a family, so we suggest a minimum of four telephone calls during each assessment phase. We typically use six calls (three per week) in our research. The measure is characterized by high retest stability and reliability (Chamberlain & Reid, 1987). We also found high con-

vergent validity of both the PDR and the CDR with other measures
of antisocial behavior (Patterson et al., 1992).

In the course of an ongoing family intervention, both the PDR
and CDR can be used to monitor change in the family and as feedback to the therapist and the family (e.g., Moore, Osgood, Larzelere,
& Chamberlain, 1994). Daily reports used as an index for monitoring intervention outcome can be administered twice weekly, scored
immediately, and graphed, not only to provide feedback on variation
in problem behavior from week to week, but also to track the re-
sponsiveness of the adolescent to interventions (see Chapter 6).

To administer the PDR and the CDR, it is ideal to have an assis-
tant make the 5- to 10-minute telephone calls. To develop rapport
with families, and to minimize confusion and scheduling problems, it
is important that the same person make all of the calls within an assessment phase. Interviewers need to be friendly but relatively task-
oriented. These interviews are not therapy, and questions relevant to
treatment should be deferred to the professional working with the
family. A polite, friendly, matter-of-fact style establishes a routine for
the interviews. These data are used to discuss cases in weekly peer supervision meetings and to discuss parental reactions to their treatment.

SCORING AND CUTOFF SCORES

A controversial issue in psychological assessment is standardization
and the use of norms. National norms, although based on large samples, do not necessarily reflect the ecology of individuals in communities or diverse minority cultures. The meaning of an assessment
may vary so dramatically that the derived scores are highly suspect.
There are two major sources of potential validity problems: the reaction of the individual to the assessment and the content of the assessment. Certainly, within the next decade, a major effort to define a
methodology for culturally sensitive measurement is needed.

We have known for some time that parenting practices vary
across ethnic groups. It is not possible to define any parenting practices as the "gold standard." Having made this point, it is important
that we mention the need to be cautious about the use of norms for
any family and to have an open discussion on these issues during the

feedback session. It is also important for all involved to remember that this is a picture at *one moment in time*, because parents may take issue with their scores as being indicative of general functioning. For therapists and researchers committed to working in a given community, we recommend assessing local families who potentially may serve as models of parenting to develop community-based norms.

As the basis of norms for our assessment battery, we selected a sample of 120 normative multiethnic families (African American, Hispanic American, American Indian, and European American) living in an at-risk urban community, who had children who were successful in middle school. Success was defined as earning grades higher than a C average, with regular attendance and no discipline contacts. Furthermore, we culled families with t scores above 65 on the externalizing scale. The risk sample consisted of youth selected based on teacher ratings of risk, including those students perceived as at risk relative to gender and ethnicity. Dishion and Bullock (2001) reported the details of the selection of the normative and high-risk samples.

The means and standard deviations for each of the protective and risk scores for child adjustment, peer influences, family context, and family management are summarized in Tables 4.1 to 4.5. As it turns out, when level of child success was controlled, there were few differences in levels of risk and protection across ethnic groups. Norms were summarized across groups, unless differences were statistically and clinically significant. To establish culturally sensitive cutoff scores, we used the minimum scores across groups. For instance, considering normative families, a mean value of 5.71 on a 10-point macrorating scale on monitoring is considered within the normative range. A cut score of 5.0 serves reasonably well for both groups; above that, parents could be considered to have enough monitoring that it is considered a protective factor.

Feedback forms are color-coded and summarized on a single page to communicate the synergistic relation between risk and protection. Risk is coded as "not present" (white), "potentially disruptive" (orange/medium gray), and as "present" (red/dark gray). Protection is scored as "needs attention" (yellow/light gray) and "present" (green/medium gray). When measures are scored, their relative magnitude can be reflected on the feedback forms by placing a letter for respondent (e.g., Y for youth, F for father, T for teacher, M for mother) in the appropriate location within the various color zones.

Given that these colors are universally represented and have similar meanings in traffic-light communication, it is likely that most parents will readily understand the meanings when provided feedback in the FCU. The idea is to communicate to parents that improving on a protective factor, especially in the family domain, will help mitigate existing concerns and risks.

We now go through each of the domains and provide a conceptual overview of the scores and demarcations of risk, leaving the details to Appendix B.

Youth Adjustment

Within the child-adjustment domain, we use the Parent Self-Check and the Youth Self-Check to score "problem behavior" and "feelings." All items are scored on a 1 to 10 scale. The problem behavior scale reflects multiple items from each measure, but "school achievement" and "feelings" are only one item. We consider this item a brief screen and supplement the information by teacher report, school observations and interviews, and intake information. Our measure of "prosocial coping" focuses on the youth report of self-control, based on the research indicating self-regulation as central in the development of problem behavior and prosocial behavior (Eisenberg, Carlo, Murphy, & Van Court, 1995; Rothbart et al., 1995). The norms for the risk and normative sample are provided in Table 4.1 from the Parent Self-Check and Youth Self-Check questionnaires.

Brief questionnaires are useful, but it is often important to provide a more comprehensive assessment of youth adjustment. In our clinical work, we use the CBCL, which includes parent, child, and teacher versions. The cross-informant scoring protocol allows comparison of raw scores and t scores across reporting agents. Six scores describe child psychopathology (risk factors) and three scores describe the child's competence in activities, academics, and peer relations (protective factors). Consideration of the unique perspectives of the child, parent, and teacher on both risk and protection is highly advantageous and provides clear cutoff scores for indicating risk or protection.

TABLE 4.1. Means and Standard Deviations for Parent and Youth Self-Check Questionnaires

	Normative (n = 41)		High risk (n = 23)		
	M	SD	M	SD	Effects
Problem behavior					
Parent Self-Check	9.33	0.52	7.20	1.36	S
Youth Self-Check	8.93	1.22	7.14	1.72	S, G
Family management					
Parent Self-Check	8.56	0.77	7.48	1.40	S, G (S × G)
Youth Self-Check	8.31	1.27	7.00	1.95	S

Note. S, status, risk versus normative; G, gender, male versus female.

Peer Influence

Assessment of the peer domain relies on the peer relations and social skills ratings completed by the teacher, parent, and child. Risk is defined by a score summarizing friend involvement in adolescent problem behavior and substance use. The peer relations score is basically a social-preference score consisting of an algebraic sum (percentage of youth who like the child minus the percentage of youth who dislike the child). The social preference score is an estimate of the extent to which peers accept the target child (Coie, Dodge, & Coppotelli, 1982; Peery, 1979). A positive score reflects general acceptance among the peer group, whereas a negative score indicates a tendency for rejection.

We assume that general acceptance by peers is a protective factor: Perceptions of acceptance among peers by teachers, parents, and youth suggest that efforts by adults to involve youth in positive social activities involving prosocial youngsters would be successful. Table 4.2 provides a summary of the means and standard deviations on the two indices of peer adjustment.

Family Context

We focus on risk factors when examining family context, using measures with preexisting norms primarily for assessment of parent depression (Radloff, 1977) and life events (Holmes & Rahe, 1967). In

TABLE 4.2. Means and Standard Deviations for Parent, Teacher, and Youth Ratings of Peer Relations

	Normative ($n = 75^a$)		High risk ($n = 23^a$)		
	M	SD	M	SD	Effects
Peer relations					
Teacher	2.83	1.32	0.65	2.33	S
Parent	2.82	1.22	1.22	2.32	S
Child[a]	2.89	1.53	2.62	1.77	S
Deviant peers					
Teacher	1.55	0.54	2.49	0.66	S
Parent	1.48	0.47	1.90	0.75	S, G (S × G)
Child	1.76	0.77	1.88	0.86	S

Note. S, status, risk versus normative; G, gender, male versus female.
[a] Normative teacher, $n = 35$, and parent, $n = 101$.

addition, we use the Dyadic Adjustment Scale (Spanier, 1976) and the Family Events Checklist (FMEVE; Fisher, Fagot, & Leve, 1998). The FMEVE provides internal (i.e., conflict and tension) and external family stress scores (i.e., daily hassles). We also have a general measure of parental substance use.

Because patterns of substance use are complex, we have a more flexible interpretation of substance use as a risk factor. For example, a parent with an extensive history of drug abuse, even though abstinent for the previous 2 months, still presents a family risk factor and may be scored in the moderate-risk range. The norms on the normative and high-risk samples are shown in Table 4.3.

Family Management

The macroratings of family management are the major protective factors within the family. The summary scores include family relationships, encouragement, limit setting, monitoring, problem solving, and drug-use norms. If there are two parents in the family, it is possible to derive separate scores. It may be advisable, however, to score the parenting team with a single measure, in order to communicate the importance of teamwork in parenting and to avoid playing into ongoing arguments between adults about who is to blame for the youth's adjustment difficulties. The means and standard deviations

TABLE 4.3. Means and Standard Deviations on Family Context Assessments

	Normative		High risk		
	M	SD	M	SD	Effects
Father	(*n* = 68)		(*n* = 11)		
Substance use					
Alcohol	5.34	2.53	3.90	2.47	S, E
Marijuana	1.41	1.71	1.81	1.77	G (S × G)
Hard drugs	0.07	0.18	0.00	0.00	
Smoking	1.54	5.88	9.08	12.69	S, E, G (S × G)
Depression	6.77	5.45	13.67	7.98	S (E × S)
Life events	10.40	7.95	9.42	6.47	
Family within stress	1.49	0.33	1.87	0.53	S
Family hassles	1.29	0.16	1.38	0.30	
Dyadic adjustment	90.62	13.20	78.67	19.38	S
Mother	(*n* = 95)		(*n* = 21)		
Substance use					
Alcohol	4.30	2.29	3.38	1.93	
Marijuana	0.89	1.07	1.10	1.04	G
Hard drugs	0.06	0.30	0.03	0.13	
Smoking	1.26	4.21	5.48	9.99	S
Depression	6.39	5.04	11.05	7.26	S, E
Life events	11.95	14.32	11.00	7.13	
Family within stress	1.55	0.41	1.84	0.48	S (E × G)
Family hassles	1.29	0.19	1.36	0.19	
Dyadic adjustment	90.69	15.86	84.92	16.42	E

Note. S, status, risk versus normative; G, gender, male versus female; E, ethnicity, European American versus African American.

for these measures are provided in Table 4.4. To complement the direct observation measure of family management, we ask the youth and caregivers to report on their perceptions of rules related to monitoring. We also use the House Rules Questionnaire, which provides an assessment of family rules relevant to parent monitoring (French & Weih, 1990).

Daily Report Data

The PDRs and CDRs are rescored so that "yes" responses to behavior problems are aggregated over phone calls. An average score of 1 reflects that an average of one behavior problem out of 10 was reported each time the parent was called. Table 4.5 is a comparison of the normative and high-risk samples. Youth report of problem

TABLE 4.4. Means and Standard Deviations on Measures of Family Management

	Normative		High risk		
	M	SD	M	SD	Effects
Parent report	(n = 101)		(n = 23)		
House rules	1.68	0.33	4.12	0.47	S (E × G, E × G × S)
Direct observation	(n = 100)		(n = 20)		
Family relationships	6.76	1.24	6.00	1.43	S
Encouraging growth	4.34	1.27	4.50	2.99	
Limit setting	6.02	1.59	5.59	1.28	G (S × E)
Monitoring	5.71	1.26	5.02	1.37	S, E
Problem solving	6.34	1.80	6.13	1.52	E (S × E)
Drug-use norms	6.99	1.29	6.31	1.36	S

Note. S, status, risk versus normative; G, gender, male versus female; E, ethnicity, European American versus African American.

TABLE 4.5. Means and Standard Deviations on Daily Report Measures of Problem Behavior

	Normative (n = 95)		High Risk (n = 32)	
	M	SD	M	SD
Child Daily Report				
Antisocial behavior	0.10	0.12	0.10	0.11
Substance use	0.00	0.02	0.03	0.08
Parent Daily Report				
Antisocial behavior	0.09	0.09	0.19	0.17
Substance use	0.00	0.02	0.01	0.07

behavior does not discriminate high-risk from normative youth, whereas parent report does. Of note, however, is that even in highly successful families, there is some daily occurrence of problem behaviors, which is often minor.

SUMMARY

This chapter provides an overview of an ecological assessment strategies for improving decision making, collaboration, and motivation when working with families with adolescents. The assessments in this chapter are offered as a minimum for family-based intervention services. Additional assessments are recommended, if clinically relevant.

In Chapter 5, we discuss how to use feedback on a family assessment to develop a working-case conceptualization, to develop a collaborative set with a parents, to build motivation to change, and to select interventions within a menu of intervention options.

5

The Family Feedback Session

In this chapter, we describe the process of addressing parents' concerns with the assessment results, building a case conceptualization, and supporting the parents' motivation to change. The feedback session, as a culmination of the initial contact and assessment, can be seen as both a brief intervention and a bridge to treatment. As such, the three-session Family Check-Up (FCU) is appropriate for all parents, regardless of demographic characteristics or severity of clinical problems. Parents with concerns that are normal to adolescence can benefit, as well as those in need of more intensive support or behavior change.

MOTIVATIONAL INTERVIEWING

Making significant and enduring changes in parenting practices is complex and challenging. For the parents, how best to focus their energy is often confusing. Changing routines and overlearned daily reactions to a child is difficult to initiate and maintain.

A transtheoretical model of behavior change allows for a flexible approach to design to assure intervention sensitivity to individual family circumstances (Prochaska & DiClemente, 1982). Motivation is the foundation of the change process from which all subsequent therapeutic interventions must build.

Prochaska and DiClemente (1982) found that over 90% of

smokers who quit did so without the aid of a therapist or behavior-change program. Careful examination of the process suggested "stages of change": When individuals make significant changes in behavior, they often go through a variety of emotionally oriented stages that may vary in length, from weeks to years. The first stage is contemplation (e.g., one begins to reflect on whether change is necessary). In the second stage, action is taken to make a change. For example, parents may decide that they need to monitor their son more carefully and have a family meeting to discuss strategies for better communication without the aid of a therapist. Given that action has been taken to make a life change, it is always necessary to maintain the change. This can be the most difficult phase of the behavior-change process, and if unsuccessful, perhaps the most discouraging. When an attempt at behavior change fails, the sense of discouragement may lead to a redefinition of goals, including a decision that change is not possible or worth the effort. Failure at behavior change may result in parents blaming their child for being "unchangeable," or blaming themselves for not being capable, which deepens the perceived intractability of the problem. Many parents of adolescents may have cycled through several efforts to change and have well-founded discouragement.

Motivational interviewing was designed as an intervention technique to "trigger" the behavior-change process by focusing on motivation to change (Miller & Rollnick, 2002). Drawing from a broad base of research, Miller and colleagues designed a set of procedures that provides parents with a basis for better decision making regarding the need for change (Brown & Miller, 1993; Miller, 1987, 1989; Miller & Sovereign, 1989). Motivational intervention incorporates a set of five behavior-change principles, encapsulated in the FRAMES model.

F refers to providing parents with data-based *feedback* about their behavior and the implications of that behavior for the future. *R* stands for communicating to clients their *responsibility* for the behavior-change process. *A* reflects the need for sound *advice* from an expert on developmental and behavior change issues. For example, in making life changes, it is often helpful to have expert advice about where the efforts should be focused, or how to take realistic steps to promote success in the behavior-change process. *M* means that, rather than providing parents with a single behavior-change option (e.g., family therapy or inpatient drug abuse treatment), it is essential that a *menu* of behavior change options be developed. Actively participating in deciding an optimal behavior-change strategy is self-motivating. *E* refers to the need to express *empathy* for the parent's situation. A classic finding in psychotherapy is the need for acceptance, support, and empathy in the behavior-change process (Rogers, 1957). Therapists must cultivate understanding and compassion for a variety of circumstantial and cultural experiences presented by parents who are considering healthy changes. Finally, the *S* in FRAMES means that parents should leave the motivational interview with a sense of *self-efficacy.* One of the best ways to promote self-efficacy is to collaborate with parents in selecting behavior-change goals that are realistic, measurable, and under their control.

The FRAMES model provides the basis for the FCU. The three-session intervention includes an intake interview, a thorough assessment, and a feedback session with the parents and, possibly, with the adolescent. The FCU was designed to (1) target parents' motivation to maintain current parenting practices that are important for young adolescents' adjustment, (2) reduce interactions that are likely to undermine the parent–child relationship or exacerbate behavior problems, and (3) increase parenting behaviors that promote adjustment and competence. The FCU can complement more extensive family therapy or stand alone for parents who choose to implement family change under their own leadership.

THE FEEDBACK PROCESS

Much of the work in conducting an effective feedback occurs away from the family. The FAsTask provides information on key parenting behaviors. Therefore, it is important for the family therapist to view carefully, as well as rate, the videotaped family interactions. At this time, it is helpful to locate sections of videotape that illustrate the parents' strengths and an interaction sequence that was troublesome and relevant to the parental concerns. Additionally, scoring the questionnaires and organizing the feedback into an understandable format should occur before meeting with the family.

If you have the good fortune to work with one or more therapists, it is extremely important to present complex or challenging cases (after scoring the data and studying the videotape) to get professional input regarding the best approach to take for each family. The comprehensive assessment and a solid case conceptualization maximize the impact of the feedback process. We now discuss the elements of case conceptualization and the feedback process itself.

Case Conceptualization

Four elements provide the organizing principles for case conceptualization: (1) the centrality of parenting to the child's success and well-being, (2) harm reduction, (3) tailoring feedback, and (4) supporting motivation to change. Within these elements, parenting is central to the long-term effort to promote success and well-being in young adolescents.

First, it is helpful to frame assessment results in terms of implications for potential interventions and support services (e.g., parent groups, family therapy). Marital problems, family transitions, health issues, and so forth, are discussed in terms of their impact on parenting practices and family communication processes.

In thinking about the prevention or reduction of problem behavior, keep in mind the catalytic role of peers in the escalation process. Our research has consistently shown the centrality of monitoring in moderating the effects of peers. In this respect, focusing on family factors that serve as a barrier to parental involvement and monitoring will be of long-term value in limiting the potential negative influence of peers. Of course, there are interdependencies in families. A strong relationship, positive limit-setting practices, encouragement, and problem solving all serve to strengthen monitoring. In the feedback process, attention to all family management practices will help build protective parenting practices.

The second principle guiding case conceptualization is harm reduction. When families are distressed, and their assessment data indicate several areas of difficulty, it is important to adopt a harm reduction perspective. This means that some time is required to consider the optimal "next-step" advice in order to control damage that is secondary to pathological processes, such as divorce-related conflict, parental drug abuse, a death in the family, a runaway child, or physical or sexual abuse. When serious problems such as these occur, the feedback process then changes to focus on the next step to reduce future harm to the child, parent, or other family members. Improvements in parenting practices, the child's behavior, or other goals are put aside in favor of creating a safe, stable family environment in which harm is eliminated or at least minimized. For instance, in the event of severe conflict and the potential for an adolescent to run away, harm reduction focuses on making the changes necessary to keep the family together. When severe school difficulties occur, the focus may be on keeping a high-risk student from being expelled.

Tailoring the feedback to the individual family is the third element of case conceptualization. Our discussion has already covered the importance of identifying larger, contextual family issues that counterindicate the parents' ability to respond to specific detailed feedback. In this situation, the feedback forms can be modified to summarize information to help the parents digest the feedback and focus on the keys issues. For example, in giving feedback in the Child Behavior Checklist, it may be helpful to summarize the individual clinical scales into the two broadband scales, externalizing and internalizing behaviors.

The fourth element of case conceptualization and feedback is supporting motivation. The goal is that parents walk away from the feedback interview feeling motivated to continue with their strengths and empowered to address their needs. During the case conceptualization process, an important goal is identifying current strengths in the parenting system. Similar to our suggested praise-to-correction ratio, a 4:1 proportion of strengths (protective factors) to concerns (risk factors) should be the goal. Even in the most difficult family circumstances, parental follow-through with the FCU process can be emphasized as a positive indication of concern for their child and a commitment to change.

The feedback forms are to be completed when you examine the assessment results within each of the broad domains: family influences, peer influences, child competencies, and problem behavior. Where entries are placed on these sheets should be based on your case conceptualization and the ratio of risk-to-protective factors. You may find it helpful to assess first the strengths within each domain, then to enter into the areas of concern, keeping a ratio of four positive feedback points to one area of concern. When formulating your strategy for giving feedback, think about the three or four (maximum) major points you want the parents to recall from the feedback session.

The Feedback Session

The feedback session can be divided into four phases. The first phase is an opportunity for parents to discuss their own self-assessment, based on their experiences in the assessment process. The second phase is clarification and support. When parents discuss their self-assessment, this is an opportunity to (1) appreciate their approach to behavior change, (2) assess their level of insight, (3) learn more about the dynamics of the family, and (4) discover issues not covered in the assessment. The third phase focuses on summarizing feedback to families, based on the information they provide. Finally, the therapist and the parents work collaboratively to develop a menu of options for improving family life and promoting the success of the child. The entire feedback session is best thought of as the beginning of a work in progress, and the final outcome will reflect a parent-guided process of interaction with the therapist.

PHASES OF THE FEEDBACK SESSION

Self-Assessment

The feedback process begins with something like the following:

> "Many parents feel like they learned something about their family after going through the assessment. Did you learn anything new? Did you think of things that might be related to some of the concerns you have for Roman?"

The majority of families bring up at least one key issue on which the therapist intends to provide feedback. Parents often perceive this question as a request to self-disclose deficits in parenting. Your response can help reframe this perception from a deficit to a goal. How the parents respond allows you to appreciate their approach to behavior change.

> "We learned that we get caught up in arguing no matter what we talk about."

This comment is enough to go on, and is the parents' first step toward making family changes. If a parent notices the arguing, chances are, you were already planning on giving her feedback on that issue. This parent will be receptive to feedback on arguing and, in fact, their insight into their difficulties can be supported.

In contrast, a parent who blames her communication problems on another family member presents a somewhat different motivational stance:

"Yeah, you can see why we never get anywhere. I've told John a thousand times that if he flunks high school, he'll never get a job. He thinks he knows everything!"

This mom's view was not changed by the assessment session, nor did she see her own lecturing and "nattering" as remotely related to the problem. It is better for you to know this now rather than after you have recommended several meetings focused on communication and wonder why your brilliant suggestions are met with stone silence.

Support and Clarification

The therapist now begins the support and clarification process. Assuming this is a one-parent family, you might proceed as follows:

"So you've targeted arguing as something that interferes with good relations. I saw that, too, when I watched your family discussion. We see arguing a lot in families with children this age. You're right, it often feels like the problems get worse when you talk about them, and the arguing gets out of control. The positive side of arguing is that it indicates your family cares about how issues get solved."

Feedback

The support and clarification phase can be a brief transition into feedback, accomplishing two goals: supporting the parent's activity in the meeting and supporting self-assessment efforts. With this information, you can clarify misconceptions about the feedback process or the goals of the meeting. A possible transition would be as follows:

"The arguing problem is solvable, and we'll see how the information you gave guides us to some ideas.

"There are a lot of changes children go through as they move into adolescence. Many families have found it useful to have the opportunity for this check-up. One way you can think of this is as getting blood pressure or temperature reports in different areas of Roman's life.

"You have a picture of how Roman is doing right now. You also know what you're doing that supports positive adjustment, which may help you sort behaviors you want to be concerned about from those that are just part of adolescence. We'll be looking for two things—what's protecting Roman against risk, and what may be putting him at risk for serious behavior problems, including substance use. You probably noticed that we asked a lot of questions about Roman's behavior and your family's current situation and style of getting along.

"I also gathered some information from Roman's teacher about his peer relations and behavior at school. This will give us a good understanding of how Roman is doing right now.

"First, we'll start with what you and the teacher reported about Roman's behavior. . . . "

The feedback phase is relatively straightforward. However, this is a lot of information for the parent to receive all at once. The therapist and parent should be sitting next to each other to allow for mutual examination of the assessment results and to reduce the potentially confrontational nature of receiving feedback.

It is best to have only one copy of the feedback forms, so that you can emphasize feedback points strategically. For example, when problems are severe, it is helpful to summarize the findings from several measures into one point.

"As you can see (*pointing to parent and teacher CBCL scores*), there's generally good agreement between you and the teacher that Roman's behavior and adjustment are a problem right now, both in terms of how he's affected, and how he's affecting others."

This draws the parent's attention to the larger issue of adjustment, as opposed to going over each individual scale, which can be punishing when they are all in the risk or needs-improvement range. Remember that many parents will be overwhelmed by the mere process of receiving feedback on issues as personal as being a parent. It is necessary to show respect for the parents' perspective and to explain that the assessment results should be considered in the context of the family's cultural and environmental situation. To communicate this, you can stop at strategic points and simply ask:

"Does this information fit with how you've been seeing the problem? When we talked before, you focused on your difficulties with Roman at home, but we didn't talk as much about school. Do you know much about the kinds of friends he hangs out with at school? Does this surprise you?"

Do not assume an understanding. Show respect and select questions that reveal information for designing a menu of change options that are helpful to the family. Be sure to monitor continually the parent's affect and reaction to information, and take time to support, validate, and put the parent at ease.

"I've just given you a lot of information. Are you having any thoughts or reactions you want to bring up?"

A contextual issue that often arises in two-parent families is marital problems. When this occurs, there are often divergent levels of satisfaction, which is usually not a surprise to the couple. However, some couples may not have discussed their marriage in some time. This is obviously a very sensitive situation that requires attention. Ignoring the marital problem may mean ignoring the source of family difficulty and may have long-term negative effects on a young adolescent's positive adjustment by virtue of contributing to an atmosphere of poor communication. Therefore, it is absolutely necessary to be direct but sensitive:

"I want to draw your attention to how each of you report your satisfaction with your marriage, because there was some disagreement there. Marian, you reported that, at this time, you're really satisfied with how things are going, and John reports being pretty unhappy with the way things are. Is this new information, or have you talked about this before?"

It is difficult to know how this will go beforehand, but it is extremely rare that serious dissatisfaction by one member of a couple has gone completely unnoticed. If it has, the information could be upsetting and arouse emotion. It is important to acknowledge and support the couple around this issue, but don't turn the feedback meeting into a marital session, because you are attempting to build momentum toward a menu of change options for the well-being of the child. Obviously, for this couple, marital therapy would be one such option within the menu.

Go through the entire feedback process and reflect on the parents' reactions, ideas, and perceptions. Communicate the importance of collaboration and that you are there to share your expertise in children and family influences. This process establishes the foundation for the next step, which is developing a menu of intervention activities.

Menu of Change Options

Consistent with the FRAMES model for motivational interviewing, parents are more likely to consider change when there is a choice of intervention options. The menu is derived in collaboration with the parents. Two items are needed on all menus. One is *doing well, no intervention needed.* Any additional comments are best worded in positive terms, such as, "Continue spending time with Nina, checking in on her homework," or "Wait one term to determine if the program she's in is working."

The other option is to have a follow-up feedback session with the teen present. This is useful for generating menu options, directing the teen toward change, and sharing the family assessment results in a motivational format. It is important that this option be directed by the parents. In families in which things are going well, a joint feedback session may be suggested to the parents as good validation for all the positive things the parents and child are doing. The joint feedback has proven to provide a positive family experience as opposed to the typical problem-focused family meetings with therapists.

A framework for developing intervention options can be found in Chapter 6. The items of this "menu" include self-change, one to two consultation sessions with the family on a specific issue (e.g., problem solving and communication), a 12-session family management group, individual family therapy, and comprehensive case management. In building a viable menu, knowledge of the school and community resources is needed. Again, the resources with which you should have expertise are those that support family management and reduce barriers to good parenting. For instance, if there is difficulty monitoring a child's daily behavior at school, a home–school communication system (card or telephone calls) would be an option on the menu.

"OK, an area we identified as a concern for you, and that also showed up as a problem in the assessment, is Nina's work and behavior at school. One option many parents find helpful is our home telephone calls. This involves a daily or weekly telephone call to you to give you specific information about Nina's assignments, homework completion, and her behavior at school.

"To prepare for these calls, we should meet twice to develop an incentive system to make this work for you at home. Does that sound like an option you might want to consider? You don't have decide now. We can just add it to the list."

When developing a menu of intervention options, it is helpful to have a writing board, so that both you and the parent can list and erase options as the discussion proceeds. Your role is first to model brainstorming for generating options, then, in the final stages of the feedback session, to promote discussion of the pros and cons of each option.

When a list of menu options is generated, you might ask the parent to select one or more for consideration.

"That's a good list we came up with. More ideas may come to you in the next week. If so, give me a call, if there's a way I can help. Do you have an idea right now of what you'd like to try?"

At times, when the parental concerns are rather serious, and when there are two parents in the family, they may wish to consider and decide the options privately. This is a process to be encouraged; however, it is important to set a time when you can call and find out what the parents have decided. It also may be possible to schedule another meeting to proceed with the next step. We encourage feedback sessions with the adolescent, if there is interest. For example:

"We didn't include Roman in this meeting, because I find it's most helpful to families if I meet with parents first, then talk with the teen. How would you prefer to discuss these results with Roman? You can do this yourself, we can discuss them with him together, or I can talk with him individually."

In this way, the parents continue to be supported in the leadership role, while also promoting open communication and support for the adolescent. A variety of strategies exist, depending on the circumstances of the case, the interest of the adolescent, and clinical conceptualization. The minimal level of feedback is sharing the results of the family discussion. More intensive levels would be a motivational interview for the adolescent, using the assessment to build motivation to change. The Youth Self-Check (similar to the Parent Self-Check) has been created to be part of the assessment battery and can be used as a central piece of your discussion.

You should finalize the FCU with a formal written report. Appendix A provides guidelines for writing an FCU report that summarizes the assessment results and supports the parents' efforts to seek services for their family.

SUMMARY

The stages-of-change model and motivational interviewing were used in the design of the FCU, in general, and the feedback session, in particular. The primary goal is using data, expert advice, empathy, and a realistic menu of change options to support the parents' decision-making process regarding the need to change.

Case conceptualization is the first step in providing feedback, which occurs before the parents arrive at the session. The feedback process is divided into four phases, including an opportunity for the parent to self-assess, and for the therapist to support and clarify the parent's self-assessment and original behavior-change goals; the feedback phase, which involves going over the assessment results collaboratively with parents; and finally, the exploration of a behavior change menu.

The next part provides a more detailed discussion of the major intervention strategies that comprise interventions within the menu that focus on addressing family management.

PART III

Implementing
a Family-Centered Menu

In this part, we discuss a variety of strategies for working with families of adolescents to improve family relationships and management. In Chapter 6, we describe our model for working individually with families, including a range of interventions from brief, focused strategies for improving a single-family management practice to more comprehensive behavioral family therapy. Chapter 7 describes family-centered interventions that are directly to the individual adolescent. Chapter 8 discusses the importance and possible cost-effectiveness of working with parents in groups.

The basic assumption underlying this section is that a variety of approaches are necessary when working with families with adolescents. Keep in mind that the interventions described in this section are selected based on a comprehensive psychosocial assessment and by virtue of a collaborative interaction with parents in a feedback interview. The interventions are "indicated" in the sense that the focus and the change venue are empirically determined. However, families may not be "indicated" from a clinical perspective, because the adolescents may not clearly meet one or more diagnostic categories, such as substance abuse or conduct disorder.

CHANGE MECHANISM

Developmental and prevention theorists agree that it is critical to understand the change mechanism (Dodge, 1993; Kellam, 1990). In our initial study, we hypothesized that family management skills would reduce the level of coercive conflict in the family, which in turn would result in fewer behavior problems outside the home (see Dishion & Andrews, 1995; Dishion, Patterson, & Kavanagh, 1992). To test this hypothesis, we looked at the change process for the families who participated in the FMC (n = 109). All families were assessed before and after participation, using direct observation of parent–child interactions and teacher ratings of antisocial behavior (Child Behavior Checklist; Achenbach, 1992). We computed simple change scores by subtracting the termination scores from the baseline scores for child and mother coercion, and teacher ratings of antisocial behavior.

Inspection of Table III.1 shows that changes (reductions or increases) in parent–child coercion over 3 months were associated with changes in teacher ratings of antisocial behavior at school. Multiple regression analyses were used to determine whether the mother changes or the child changes were most predictive of change in antisocial behavior. The results of this analysis are presented in Figure III.1. Child changes in negative interaction were the most predictive of change in behavior in the school context. However, changes in observed mother and child behavior were highly correlated (r = .61), showing that the coercive interaction between the parent and child is critical for change.

TABLE III.1. Correlated Change of Parent–Child Coercion and Teacher Ratings of Externalizing Behavior

	Month		
	1	2	3
1. Child coercion	1.00		
2. Mother coercion	0.61*	1.00	
3. Teacher ratings	0.33*	0.24*	1.00

* $p < .05$.

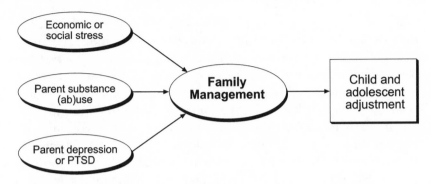

FIGURE III.1. Family management as a mediator of family context.

Support exists for the hypothesis that improved family management results in reduced parent–child conflict and improved behavior in other settings, as indicated by teacher ratings at school. When working with families, it is important to keep an eye on coercive interchanges.

INTENSITY OF THE INTERVENTION

There is reason to be skeptical when thinking that a linear dose–response relationship exists between the amount of therapist contact and the level of change in families. As of the present writing, no clear relationship surfaces between the number of sessions and changes in coercive interactions (Stormshak & Dishion, 2002; Weber, 1998). However, in a study of clinical archives of 90 families involved in behavioral family therapy, we found that two-thirds of the families did make clinically significant changes (Dishion & Patterson, 1992). The next question arises: How much intervention is needed for families?

We looked at this issue for parents who participated in our FMC-based groups. In defining clinically significant change, we used the strategy outlined by Jacobsen and Truax (1991), and formulated two groups from the family management program participants. The first group was distressed at baseline and made clinically significant improvements in observed coercive behavior at termination. The second group was also distressed at baseline but did not exhibit clinically significant change. Parents were called weekly and asked about their child's antisocial behavior and substance use. The observations were aggregated into 4-week periods. Figure III.2 shows that those families who made clinically significant changes experienced reductions in problem behavior by the fourth to fifth group meeting.

It is safe to say that the selection of strategies for working with families, in general, will reflect their level of distress, as indicated in the assessment. Often, we find a general correlation between the level of distress, developmental history, and seriousness of the problem behavior, and the intensity and duration of the family management therapy. However, even though this is true, therapists working with families need to understand what we know about the change process in order to keep attuned to indicators that the interventions are indeed helpful to the family and adolescent. Also, the form and intensity of work with a family may change over time, because response to intervention itself can be a diagnostic indicator. A reactive response to an intervention that leads to a deteriorating family situation (e.g., revealed abuse, divorce) serves as an indicator that a brief intervention strategy may need to evolve into more intensive support.

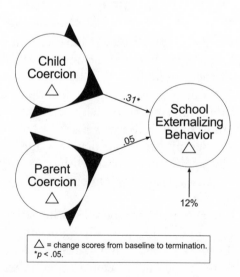

FIGURE III. 2. Change in coercion and change in adolescent problem behavior.

6

Interventions
for Family Management

In this chapter, we discuss a menu of parent interventions that promote family management. We propose that a variety of change options be made available to parents in the form of an intervention menu, based on the FMC. The menu includes individual meetings with parents on specific parenting issues (e.g., communication), periodic telephone calls, school monitoring service, brief therapy (two to three sessions), a parent group (see Chapter 8), or family management therapy (six or more sessions).

The therapy process, as it applies to working with parents, is reviewed, as well as strategies for promoting change in family management. The FCU has set the foundation for this active phase of the change process. Therapist attention and skill facilitate the parents' and family's agreements with the change strategy selected.

THERAPY PROCESS

A frequent assumption underlying parenting intervention programs is that parents want to be taught parenting skills. Whereas it is probably true that most parents do want to improve their relationship with their child, compliance with any behavior-change routine is inherently difficult. Lessons from research on medical prescriptions are particularly instructive: People, as a rule, do not follow medical regimens (Sackett, 1979). A reasonable assumption is that the more habitual the parental behavior pattern, the more noncompliant the parents are with treatment. For example, Miller (1989) reported that the more addictive the behavior, the fewer the attempts at making behavioral change. Given the stability of antisocial behaviors across time, it makes sense to consider the family and peer interaction patterns within which they are embedded as relatively habitual and intractable.

Commitment and follow-through with the change process are challenging. Difficulty in the change process may, in part, also be a function of the parent population. The uncooperative spirit of parents of children with oppositional and conduct disorder has been widely acknowledged. O'Dell (1982) surveyed 16 parent-training therapists and found that only 27% of the families they saw were considered easy to treat. Moreover, parents of teenagers may have less enthusiasm about change than do parents of younger children. Parents of older children have a longer history of difficulty; therefore, they have less motivation and fewer expectations for success. Not surprisingly, Dishion and Patterson (1992) found that parents of older children were more likely to drop out of treatment compared to parents of younger children. Families of older children who remained in treatment, however, changed equally.

In the early 1980s, our colleagues at the Oregon Social Learning Center began to study intensively the role of therapists and parents in the change process (Chamberlain, Patterson, Reid, & Kavanagh, 1984; Patterson & Chamberlain, 1994; Patterson & Forgatch, l985). First, a coding system was built for therapist behavior (Chamberlain et al., 1984), to allow the study of the sequential process of therapeutic interaction and to identify the ability of each person in the therapy setting to alter behavior.

These studies revealed that, paradoxically, therapists who exerted their expertise in sessions with parents actually elicited "resistance" to change. In a series of single-subject reversal design experiments (i.e., ABAB), therapist use of *teach, confront, support*, and *reframe* were experimentally manipulated (Patterson & Forgatch, l985). Increases in therapist *teach* and *confront* led to an increase in parent resistance. Similarly, Miller, Benefield, and Tonigan (2001) found significant covariation between parent arguing, interrupting, and being off-task, and therapist use of confrontation. Collectively, these findings suggest that resistance to change can be elicited inadvertently by therapist behavior and is not necessarily a personality trait of the parent.

It is also true that resistant parents can wear down therapists (Patterson & Forgatch, 1985). Therapists become discouraged and less motivated when working with resistant parents, just as marital partners become less interactive with their depressed spouses (Biglan, Lewin, & Hops, 1990; Hops et al., 1990). One of the most important functions of weekly therapy supervision meetings is to provide support for the efforts of each therapist who engages in the struggle of behavior change with parents.

CHALLENGES TO FAMILY CHANGE

Table 6.1 summarizes some of the common therapy process dynamics that can emerge in the course of behavior change. These are organized to reflect the impact of family patterns on therapist reactions and possible solutions.

Although there are more than three types of dynamics the thera-

TABLE 6.1. Common Therapy Process Dynamics in Family Change

Therapy process dynamic	Behavioral sign	Therapist reactions to minimize	Therapeutic solutions
Enmeshment/ negative sentiment override	Blames adolescent, "bad seed," "nothing works with him or her," or "I won't!"	Defensive, confrontive	Validate, video feedback, reframe, problem solve, explore content
Avoids problems and/ or neglectful	Unmotivated, passive, disengaged, "I can't"	"Parenting the parent"	Small steps, positive change strategies, incentives for engagement
Cultural disconnect	Lack of trust, cancels, quits	Avoidance of contact	Show respect, query, sensitivity training, bicultural training diversity in therapy team

pist may experience when working with families, those shown in Table 6.1 are quite common and often require attention. The FCU provides the advantage of a preview of these dynamics before engaging in the active intervention stage. We hypothesize that an advantage of the FCU is that the change dynamic of the parent may be anticipated and addressed initially, thereby improving the efficiency in the active intervention stage. As reported in Chapter 10, we find moderate effect sizes for high-risk adolescents with an average of 10 sessions over 3 years (Dishion, Kavanagh, Schneiger, Nelson, & Kaufman, 2002).

Negative Emotion

High levels of negative emotion in the change process actually suggest investment. If parents do not care about the adolescent, it is unlikely that they will engage in the change process or bother to resist change efforts. In this sense, the parents' investment can be a positive prognostic sign for change. However, parents can be emotionally invested toward a negative end such as showing a partner or a professional that the adolescent has "negative intentions." This investment, then, is toward getting the adolescent out of the family.

Therapists know they are dealing with this type of investment if their own reactions are toward defining a family member as the problem or confronting parents about their attitude toward the adolescent. Behavioral signs in the parent include blaming and statements that suggest that the adolescent is a "bad seed" (i.e., "He's just like his father."). This process in marriages has been referred to as "negative sentiment override" (Weiss et al., 1996). The idea is that the negative feelings within a relationship completely override the potential for experiencing positive family interactions. If parents with negative sentiment override do not feel that the therapist is supporting their attitude, they may become resistant to therapist suggestions and support, reducing the potential for a therapeutic alliance.

Positive strategies for redirecting this negative emotional energy include looking for opportunities to validate the parents' emotional experience, without supporting their negative attributions. A stepfather who is frustrated with difficult adolescent behavior, and whose wife is insensitive to his experience, might be moved from a negativistic stance if his experience is understood and appreciated, for instance:

"I can see you're at your wit's end. It must seem like you're between a rock and a hard place sometimes. It's tough being a stepparent, because you sometimes end up being seen as the bad
guy."

Such a statement, in the right situation, can open the door for a
deeper understanding within the marriage, and perhaps for better
family communication.

To work with negative emotion in family dynamics, it is extremely important that the therapist gain a stance of "objectification," in other words, to be seen as a professional whose observation could be of benefit. Videotaped feedback is a useful tool for
working through the emotionally enmeshed situation. It is often
helpful to review with a parent a videotape of his interaction with his
teenager, to explore his own emotions during specific interchanges.
Often, it is difficult for the parent to see his own emotional reactions.
In a supportive context, watching himself on video can be a powerful
statement that requires few words. The therapist is then in the position of validating, listening, reflecting, and labeling the negative emotion dynamic for future problem solving.

Neglect and Avoidance

Parents can neglect or avoid their youth a variety of ways. In working with adolescent problem behavior, perhaps the most common example is the sibling–parent dynamic (Patterson, 1982). Most parents
prefer never to set limits with their child. Setting limits can feel bad
or temporarily cause distance in the parent–child relationship. For
parents who are emotionally vulnerable, this distance may be too
much for them to handle. Adolescents may become punitive when a
parent attempts to set limits for the first time, or parents may neglect
their adolescent, unaware of dangerous or troublesome situations in
which setting limits is critical. Such parents may come across as passive in the therapy process, which may make the therapist want to
"parent the parent."

In most situations, however, the fundamental dynamic is not addressed. The parent eventually needs to become more active in parenting, if the changes he seeks are to be realized. Again, the assessment and feedback sessions can be used to explore the lack of
motivation this style represents. In addition, the change process can

begin with small steps that support the parent in a leadership role. Parents' successful implementation of an incentive program can be enough to empower them to further assume the parenting role.

Beginning with areas of strength is an excellent way to help the neglectful parent become more engaged actively in parenting. To begin, it may be useful simply to contract with the parent to spend more recreational time with the teenager in activities that are intrinsically interesting to both. For example, to build a more positive relationship between an adolescent daughter and her father, we developed a contract for the dad to pick her up from school on his way home from work.

For programs that provide services to parents who struggle with more severe distractions and disruptions in parenting, it may be necessary to provide incentives for engagement. This has been referred to as the *community reinforcement approach*. In the area of drug addiction treatment, parents are provided with incentives for periods of sobriety (Budney, Higgins, Delaney, Kent, & Bickel, 1991; Fleischman, 1979; Higgins et al., 1993). As applied to parenting, we offer incentives for participation and attendance to parenting groups, salaries for engaging in family management therapy (Fleischman, 1979), and school incentives for engaging in the family interventions (e.g., schools will often agree not to expel a student if the parent attends a parent group or other parenting service).

Cultural Disconnect

A serious therapeutic process problem can result from a cultural disconnect between the therapist and the family. This problem stems from the inability of the therapist to read and to be sensitive to parent experiences because of a lack of exposure to the family's cultural background and history.

Interventions with parents must be culturally sensitive (Kumpfer et al., 1996). Programs developed primarily with one cultural-ethnic group are likely to be culturally insensitive. Minority-group members with a history of maltreatment from mental health or social service agencies will be distrustful of any intervention that does not respect and support cultural differences in parenting practices (Duran & Duran, 1995). Families, as well as therapists, experiencing the stress of acculturation need expertise and support that is sensitive to various cultural perspectives (Coatsworth, Szapocznik, Kurtines, &

Santisteban, 1997). At times, the content of the intervention may require adaptation to the family's culture. Parents might not attend parent training programs, or often, they drop out prematurely, feeling hopeless about their potential for having an impact on their child (Dishion & Patterson, 1992). A rigid, culturally narrow intervention program is unlikely to support the unique challenges of minority parents (Szapocznik et al., 1980) and could lead to low use and engagement in intervention resources (Sue, Bingham, Porche-Burke, & Vasquez, 1999).

The parents' sense that a service is oriented around the needs and assumptions of another culture is understandably a disincentive to engagement. In the best scenarios, parents openly express a lack of trust, or worse, they find a way to avoid the service. In fact, it is probably in the best interest of the family to avoid mental health services that are insensitive, because more harm than good can result from another well-intentioned "professional" who is ignorant of the strengths of diverse parenting practices, or to the historical and social context of service delivery in the minority community. At times it may be tempting to avoid contact with parents with whom there is a cultural disconnect.

The same dynamic that serves as a barrier to engaging in majority-culture mental health services may undermine the parenting, especially for recently immigrated families. Differential acculturation within families can undermine parents' ability to influence their adolescents' lives. Hispanic families, for example, may experience stress secondary to the adolescent assuming the cultural values of the majority culture. Respectful queries into the parents' experiences with school personnel and other professionals can often unveil repeated misunderstandings that should be avoided in the future.

Parental reaction to the assessment may help the therapist understand parenting values. At a minimum, the therapeutic team (therapist supervision group) should represent cultural expertise, in order to avoid cultural bias in the delivery of services. Showing respect for those values helps tremendously in establishing a collaborative relationship.

Questions about the adolescent and parents' experiences in the community also may reveal historical or recent events that affect parenting and adolescent behavior. For instance, when working with some American Indian families, it is critical to be aware of the impact of boarding schools on parenting practices and the collective trauma of the community (Duran & Duran, 1995). Sensitivity to cultural and historical factors avoids the potential of undermining a family's sense of ethnic identity and cultural pride, and enhances the collaborative relationship. A shared understanding of the cultural issues facing a family can go a long way toward providing context for bicultural training, which may promote the family's functioning more effectively in the majority community (Coatsworth et al., 1997; Szapocznik et al., 1988).

STRATEGIES FOR SUPPORTING CHANGE

In addition to these therapy process issues, a number of basic principles are endorsed by virtually all effective interventions with families (Henggeler et al., 1998; Webster-Stratton, 1992). These principles apply when working with parents across a variety of therapeutic contexts.

A Shared Perspective

The goal of family management therapy is *not* that the family accepts the therapist's perspective, but that there is a *shared* perspective between the therapist and parent. Although we may know that certain parent–child interaction patterns are significant in the etiology of antisocial behavior, the parent is less likely to see the problem this way. Any form of intervention work requires equal consideration of the family's story, in addition to the therapist's perspective. This creates an optimal condition for parental action and the development of the skills needed to maintain change. The first step is sharing these perspectives.

A Collaborative Set

Because of the strong empirical base underlying most behavioral parent training, therapists usually have a predetermined set of skills they want parents to learn. Put more simply, much of parent training can be characterized by the therapist knowing what parents need to do, then telling them how to do it (Chamberlain et al., 1984). Unfortunately, this establishes a hierarchical relationship, with the therapist as the expert and little room for parent ownership of the change process (Webster-Stratton & Herbert, 1993).

Helping people make a change is a matter of first having a relationship that allows us to influence their thinking and behavior. We do not believe that this comes from being an "expert." Taking this role may get the family's attention initially but doesn't ensure that they will accept the skills or try to implement them. The basis for developing collaboration is creating a problem-solving focus that involves everyone in the solution. It also helps define the roles of the family and the therapist.

Blame can be assigned to parents when the therapist sees their previous life course of antisocial behavior, school failure, or drug use played out again in their teenager. Parents are easy to blame, too, when they have backed away from parenting. It is also easy to frame the problem as the teen's rigidity in not wanting to accept guidelines that are beneficial for long-term success (e.g., doing homework or staying away from kids who use drugs). Our belief is that, as therapists, we must remind ourselves at all stages of work that problems are to be solved—they are not attached to people. This also implies that the therapist shares the problem and doesn't have the solution. Working together will bring about solutions.

Webster-Stratton and Herbert (1993) summarized collaborative models as including support, empowerment, expertise, and challenging parents to change and to predict problems and setbacks. In our parent groups, the leader stimulates the parents' discussion of family management and other family-centered issues. Work with parents is a balance between support and sharing perspectives and expertise.

Our intervention model conceptualizes parenting skills as the principal proximal determinants of adolescent problem behavior and the primary targets of intervention. Parental stress, depression, poverty, minority status, and other factors of family and community ecology are distal to the change process. This is not to dismiss the tremendous influence exerted by these factors from time to time. However, these factors are often variables over which neither the family nor the therapist has much control. Significant therapeutic resolution of these issues is unlikely.

Ecological Sensitivity

Compared to the attention paid to resistance as a trait, little attention has been given to the family ecology of resistance to change (Chamberlain et al., 1984; Miller, 1989; Webster-Stratton & Herbert, 1993). An ecological model of socialization is sensitive to the disruptive impact of poverty, minority status, divorce, unemployment, and parent psychopathology (e.g., depression and drug abuse) on parenting. Given that these experiences are disruptive, they likely underlie parental resistance to change. If therapists are insensitive to a family's context, then they may be unaware of any dynamics that might interfere with the change process.

When parenting issues are embedded within long-standing contextual disruption (e.g., divorce), the content and process of change needs to be adapted to fit the family situation. Change may be impossible until the disruption, such as a serious marital problem or parental substance abuse, is reduced. Prinz and Miller (1994) found improved outcomes in clinical trials that explored contextual issues, in addition to skills development and family management. Some common family context issues to address when working with families of adolescents emerged.

Stepfamilies

This is a commonly identified area for which parents request information or help. Even if both adults (the biological parent and the stepparent) are well-adjusted and skilled as parents, there may still be difficulties. Children do not always react to a new marital situation with the same enthusiasm as adults. Working out the stepparenting system is likely to be a struggle, even under the best of circumstances.

A proactive therapist can contribute a great deal to this situation. Certain problems are predictable, and if anticipated, may normalize parents' experiences. In this way, problems are normalized and stepparents benefit from strong communication skills and negotiated roles. We found that, in addition to brief consultations, many stepparents benefit from the family management groups, in which the entire domain of family life is discussed and negotiated in a stepwise fashion.

Marital Distress

Our experience indicates that a fair number of at-risk, two-parent families are maritally distressed and have not dealt with or discussed that issue. Marital distress has long been known to be a common dynamic of families with a troubled child. Studies of these families have led to defining the process of triangulation, in which the adolescent inadvertently serves as the lightning rod for husband–wife conflict, which unfortunately prevents the couple from identifying and solving the real problem.

Most effective approaches to solving marital stress rely on building communication skills. Therefore, an intervention that focuses on listening and negotiating conflict could certainly be helpful. It is important, however, not to naively present such a brief intervention as solving marital distress. Communication and relationship skills interventions are introduced as the first phase of work on the marital problem and may lead to a decision regarding the next step, including referrals.

Divorce

It goes without saying that divorce is disruptive to families. Moreover, the effects of an "ugly divorce" can last for years. Research clearly indicates that the major difficulty for children is being caught between two ex-spouses who are waging war against one another. Secondary to anger, parents may be unaware that they are putting the child between them, and such a process might not be revealed in the FCU (e.g., when only one parent participates). Careful interviewing and discussion is often needed to see how communication and cooperation works between two ex-spouses.

A brief intervention on the divorce theme includes a variety of focuses, one of which is emotional. For parents ravaged by the stress of coping with parenting while meeting their own emotional and social needs, emotional support may redirect discussions away from the children and, more appropriately, to adults in the parents' world. A problem-solving focus is also common. It is helpful to explore strategies of communication and conflict resolution with the caregiving parent in a way that minimizes the child being caught in the middle. Role playing, clear communication, perspective taking, and listening skills are critical to constructive problem solving with an ex-spouse.

In joint custody situations, it may be helpful to meet with both parents to discuss a system of cooperation and coparenting that works for parents *and* child. Consistency and support by both parents go a long way toward laying a foundation from which children and adults begin to heal. When joint custody is friendly, these brief consultations can be invaluable. By contrast, in situations of animosity, we suggest referral to a professional mediator.

Parental Psychopathology

Drug use and mental instability can cause serious disruption of parenting, but brief consultations in this area can provide an opening for referral service. Explore the impact on the parent, family, and child. Reflective listening and motivational interviewing can assist the parents in the decision-making process.

For several family issues, referral to more intensive services is often warranted. One advantage of referral is that it reduces the drain on the FRC staff, who, by definition, need to be engaged in a menu of services for families. The disadvantage is that parents often do not follow through on referrals, which involves establishing yet another personal relationship with an unknown professional. The more that can be done to minimize losing the family in the professional "handoff," the better. Making a call and an appointment with the parent present is one strategy to use. Another way to ensure that families connect with referral sources is to include a written report based on the FCU. Referrals for parental substance abuse, marital therapy, parental psychiatric status, or individual therapy are often recommended. However, it may be possible to work with families on these issues within the family-centered approaches.

Finding the Strengths

Identifying and using strengths is an important part of the parental sense of hope and self-efficacy, and should continue throughout the intervention process. Beginning and ending family work with an identification of strengths actually helps parents experience those strengths. This can be done in an ongoing discussion of their efforts to make change.

Drawing attention to the family's adaptation of intervention ideas also can highlight strengths. The therapist's role is to provide support to carry out changes. Expertise derived from working with families can be shared to maximize success. Advice giving is minimized and structured for answering questions, rather than teaching down to parents.

Neutralizing Negative Emotions

We previously discussed the role of coercion in adolescent problem behavior, with much attention directed toward decreasing negative emotions. Anger and upset elicit a chain of reactions, often including destructive family interactions that are essentially on autopilot. We provide the rationale that it is difficult to be planful when upset, which usually creates a condition for reacting. We talk with parents and teens about maximizing the likelihood that ideas will be heard if they are expressed in a neutral tone, yet we have met many parents and teens who have said that yelling or showing extreme reaction is the only way to get attention.

It is difficult for teens to learn from parents who are upset, and it is next to impossible to be empathic or instructive with an angry teenager.

Support through Skills Development

Like all therapists, we struggle with finding a good balance between support and skills development. Commiserating with the problems and challenges that confront many families is not difficult; however, it can prevent an objective point of view. It is helpful to support parents' efforts, even when they do not seem to be following the course we think might work best. It is equally important to provide a continuous, gentle push to help parents move toward their goals.

The best support someone can receive is to gain a new tool to cope with the problems that inevitably resurface. Both skills and support are to be used in equal proportions, and, in practice, support is experienced through the skills we offer families.

Flexibility in Delivery

Family-based interventions need to be flexible with respect to scheduling, format, content, and focus of the intervention activity. Typically, families are not inclined to participate in family interventions led by professionals, have more than a 5-week time commitment, or involve the school or other parents. Spoth and Redmond (1996) advanced the field by using marketing research strategies to understand better optimal ways of engaging and working with families. Despite these advances, not all parents seek the same intervention services, which makes it necessary to offer a wide range of intervention times and modalities in a variety of locations.

A rigid focus on parenting issues is not as effective as encompassing multiple levels of issues that disrupt parenting (Henggeler et al., 1986; Prinz & Miller, 1994). The flexibility of the intervention agenda is consistent with the principles of effective interventions for reducing alcohol problems (Miller & Rollnick, 2002). A menu of intervention options increases motivation.

THE MENU

The principles outlined here are the foundation of good process, regardless of the length or form of family intervention. Parents may begin the change process with small steps, such as watching a videotape on parenting, and later move on to seek more intensive support to change pernicious family dynamics such as coercive arguments with an adolescent, marital disharmony in parenting, avoidance of monitoring and setting limits, or poor communication practices. The kinds of issues that parents of adolescents face are relatively finite.

We consider several intervention options to be basic to the overall model.

Self-Help

Many parents simply prefer to make changes on their own. This preference could be an indication of self-sufficiency, a need for privacy, or suspicion of mental health services based on past personal experience or historical factors (Duran & Duran, 1995). It is important to honor this choice rather than attempt to guide the parents toward involvement in an intervention that they would be unlikely to follow.

It may be difficult not to push when the parental preference does not fit with the therapist's presumptions for the family. At such times, remember that it is the *parents' process of change,* and they are more likely to come to the therapist for resources in the future if he accepts their initial choice for self-change. A good compromise is asking permission to check in with the parents in a month or so, to see how things are going, and to be a resource in processing questions or clarifying concepts.

A self-help option may be available within a variety of service delivery settings. A library with videotapes, manuals, and brochures is an excellent way to support the self-change process. Webster-Stratton and colleagues (1988) found that leaderless parental groups who watched parenting videos made significant improvements in parenting practices, and their children showed reductions in behavior problems in the preschool years. Plausibly, some parenting practices, once identified as problematic, can be changed without professional support. The extent to which clinical psychology acknowledges and supports self-change is apparent when we finally establish a process in which we "give psychology away" (Sarason, 1981).

A number of excellent parenting videos are available that could be placed in an FRC library or clinic environment. We encourage you to review video resources that are relevant to the families you will be serving. This is especially important for culturally diverse populations. The FMC includes handouts and worksheets for parents that can be collated to form an individualized *parent packet*, specific to the needs of each family (Dishion et al., 2003). In addition, videotapes are available that address each major content area of the FMC. The book *Parents and Adolescents Living Together* is also an outstanding resource (Forgatch & Patterson, 1989; Patterson & Forgatch, 1985). Other self-help books on marital adjustment, stepfamilies, or depression make a good first step in the change process.

Jamie, a 14-year-old boy in his first year of high school, to date, has shown little problem behavior and has done well in school. His family was self-referred because of an extremely upsetting series of arguments between Jamie, his stepmother, and his father.

Two years earlier, Jamie's father remarried, and the newly-weds quickly had a baby girl. Life changed radically for Jamie. His stepmother was at home constantly and immediately assumed a caregiving role with Jamie. Recently, Jamie was asked to periodically baby-sit. His grades began to drop, and he became argumentative with his parents.

In the assessment, several strengths in the family were identified. By and large, these parents had positive skills but unrealistic expectations for Jamie, with respect to his needs in adapting to his new family life.

We recommended that the parents read a book on stepparenting by Visher and Visher (1979), and gave them material and a videotape on listening. We also recommended that the stepmom be less active in managing Jamie's school progress over the next 6 months, and that his father resume involvement with Jamie. The therapist called in 1 month to see if there was a need for more direct support.

Brief Family Interventions

If the family is strong on setting limits and monitoring but weak on positive approaches to behavior management, then an intervention that increases the level of positive reinforcement (incentive program) is recommended. Families that are generally strong on "control" techniques, but low on positive reinforcement usually behave that way because of their own childhood history. A structured approach to helping them support positive adolescent behavior can benefit family relationships and increase positive behavior.

Brief family therapy involves one to four sessions on specific topics that have emerged as concerns in the FCU. We propose brief consultations as an excellent strategy when family management practices are basically intact, but the family still benefits from attention to one family management area. Our general approach to designing brief interventions is hierarchical, as shown in Figure 6.1.

Adolescence represents a phase shift, with increased conflict in the parent–adolescent relationship. The first option for addressing a family difficulty is to support problem solving and communication in the parent–adolescent relationship. Those parents who effectively master this transition reorganize their interactions by providing their teenagers with appropriate levels of autonomy and input (Granic et al., 2003; Robin & Foster, 1989). The entire section on relationship building in the FMC addresses a wide range of skills that are necessary for effective parent–adolescent problem solving. If the parents can be flexible on an issue (e.g., chores, homework, curfew), then it

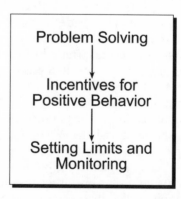

FIGURE 6.1. Hierarchical strategy for brief interventions.

is best to approach a family difficulty with a problem-solving approach.

Supporting parental interest in building or maintaining a positive relationship with their young teen is integral to the welfare of the family. This is accomplished by first establishing good listening skills, then negotiating conflict constructively, and finally, finding ways to share recreation and free time together. This has been referred to as "building the family bank account" (Dishion & Patterson, 1997; Patterson & Forgatch, 1987).

The second level in a brief intervention is to provide reinforcement for a positive adolescent behavior that "replaces" a problem behavior. This is usually straightforward, as in supporting the development of homework skills in an adolescent who is having trouble in middle or high school. A brief intervention focusing on positive behavioral support follows the RPM principle of behavior change: Realistic, under the Parents' control, and Measurable. The FMC contains handouts and a focused curriculum on applying the RPM principle to use of positive behavioral support strategies of behavior change.

For more seriously delinquent teenagers, setting limits is needed to reduce behavior that compromises safety or long-term adjustment. More serious adolescent problem behavior suggests a more intensive level of support in family management. However, at times, serious problem behavior may seem to come out of nowhere, and all that is required is for parents to upgrade their limit-setting strategies or respond to an aberrant episode of misbehavior.

> In one middle school, several eighth-grade students decided to take the day off and have a party, complete with marijuana and alcohol. Although serious, the behavior was unusual for most of the students. In response, our FRC therapist met with the parents to discuss limit setting, as well as cooperation among parents on monitoring. Two of the five families had individual sessions on setting limits with teenagers.

We proposed a systematic approach to working with parents on setting limits with adolescents. This option involves the SANE guidelines, which are briefly summarized in Figure 6.2. These guidelines outline a nonpunitive approach to setting limits that is sustainable and can be consistently followed by parents over time. Consistency in setting limits is the key to effectiveness.

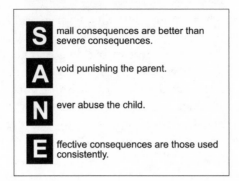

FIGURE 6.2. The SANE guidelines for parents: Setting limits.

Bill (stepfather) and Dharma (mother), who have been married for 10 years, attend church regularly with their two adolescents. Their 15-year-old son has always been a handful, having been diagnosed as "attention deficit and hyperactive" since age 5. The parents have never used medication to control his behavior.

The boy is a pleasant, well-mannered adolescent, but he is also impulsive and challenging to manage. Bill's style of discipline is more authoritarian, whereas Dharma is authoritative. Of late, they actually seem to undermine each other's efforts. Bill sets a consequence for a misbehavior, and Dharma sympathizes with their son and changes the consequence. Over the last 6 months, they have been arguing about how to set limits on their adolescent's behavior.

School Monitoring

As developmental psychologists suggest, the operating procedures of the public school environment are not conducive to success for some young adolescents (Eccles et al., 1993). Many students need more adult support to manage their daily routines and learning schedules. Parents are often unaware of this need and may be shocked to hear about problem behavior or poor academic progress *after the fact.*

Our contention is that more effort should be placed on redesigning school systems to keep youth engaged and to reduce the proliferation of alternative school environments for high-risk youth. School monitoring and encouraging parental support of positive school engagement is the key to retention of high-risk students.

School monitoring can either stand on its own as an intervention or accompany a brief intervention, family therapy, and case management. Within the FCU, the parents and therapist review the adolescent's pattern of attendance, behavior, and completion of homework assignments, as reported by teachers and school staff. Following the RPM principle, we target behavior-change goals to determine whether they are realistic for the adolescent, then work with parents to ensure that they effectively *support* positive school reports. A key principle is that we encourage parents to refrain from punishing the adolescent for negative school reports. We also establish a system of communication between the school and the parents to ensure periodic (e.g., daily, weekly) reports on behavior, attendance, and completion of school work.

Several approaches are used to establish a system of communication. One is to place the responsibility on the student for taking the "home–school card" around to teachers, then home to the parents. It is the rare adolescent who will not lose or forget this card, even when his or her intentions are positive. If the student is responsible for the card, then incentives should be provided for remembering the card, regardless of the contents of the report. Many public schools are prepared to provide such reports, and parents can call school staff to get weekly or daily information regarding, at the least, attendance, and at times, behavior and completion of homework assignments. If the therapist works in an FRC, this is an excellent service to provide parents and an excellent engagement tool. The FRC therapist collects the information and periodically communicates this to parents.

One decision for the therapist and parents to make is the frequency of reports to parents on the teen's behavior, attendance, and completion of homework assignments. Daily communication is indicated when a student is close to failing, suspension, or expulsion. If the problem is moderate, a weekly communication system is preferable. Occasionally, a parent may get two weekly reports, then move to biweekly or monthly reports. Of course, report cards serve the same function, but they are less frequent.

Isabel and her son Josh have always been alone. Isabel moved frequently when Josh was young, but now they have been in the same town for 3 years. Isabel is about to finish in architecture school, and Josh is a sophomore in high school. Although Josh is an intelligent and personable youth, he has little self-discipline and quickly disengages from the public school system. He attended only 25% of his sophomore classes, and was bound to repeat this pattern, when the family was referred.

Isabel is intimidated by Josh and can't recall ever setting a limit on his behavior. The therapist established a daily home–school card that focused on attendance. The system is simple: If Josh attends school that day, he can use his skateboard; if he doesn't attend school, the skateboard is locked in his mother's car trunk.

This contingency was enough to get the behavior-change ball rolling, and Isabel eventually supported Josh's completion of homework. He achieved passing grades in his first semester and attended the majority of the term. This was a first in his high school experience.

Parent Networking

An advantage of working within a school is the opportunity to facilitate parent problem-solving meetings. A part of being able to effectively monitor young adolescents is communication with their friends' parents, to share rules and information, and to identify places where children are getting into trouble ("hot spots"). When peer problem situations occur within the school setting, a positive strategy is to invite parents to a meeting to problem-solve together about how to keep their adolescents safe and out of trouble (e.g., fighting, peer harassment issues, or get-togethers at unsupervised homes). If a format of cooperation is established at the beginning, common parental denial and anger at other parents can be avoided. Our experience is that if parents really do not feel that it is their issue, they will not attend the meeting.

Depending on the situation, it is good to include school personnel as additional resources for strategies and information. These meetings are often the springboard for continued networking, without the need for professional facilitation.

Family Therapy and Support

The FMC can also serve as a template for individual family therapy. This involves a personal connection with the entire family and regular meetings (once a week is fine) in a confidential setting. There are several avenues of family therapy, but when working with families individually, it often helps to plan frequent, brief assessments in the home and school, so that the therapist and parents can monitor progress. Dishion and Stormshak (in press) discuss this as the AIM of behavior change: Assessment, intervention, and motivation are addressed in all phases of behavior change.

Chamberlain and Reid (1987) described the PDR and its clinical utility. We extended the PDR to include the CDR and Teacher Daily Report (TDR). The reports can be weekly or more often, but include a 24-hour recall to minimize biases due to global reports.

Family therapy with adolescents is often conducted with two therapists, one representing the parental system and another representing the perspective of the adolescent. Chapter 7 discusses in detail how to structure and organize sessions with adolescents, in order to be consistent with a family-centered perspective.

The conventional outpatient paradigm is that the family meets weekly in the clinic and proceeds through the behavior-change process until the work is completed. Again, we find that initiating the change process with the FCU shortens the number of sessions by clarifying the focus of the interventions needed and are identifying barriers to change.

Our approach to working with families is consistent with the multisystemic model for family therapy (Henggeler et al., 1998). As discussed by Dishion and Stormshak (in press), the ecological approach focuses heavily on the social interactions within the family as intervention targets. Our model differs from most intervention models in that our family therapy is initiated and guided by assessment. We prioritize our intervention targets in collaboration with the adult caregivers, taking into account the family ecology, the relationship patterns within the family, and motivation.

Consistent with a flexible approach, it may be necessary to conduct family sessions in the home and to meet frequently during the initial months of engagement. There are several advantages to having home sessions, one being that we enhance the ecological validity of the sessions by direct observations of exigencies of daily family life. Also, it may be necessary to link family interventions with existing family services (i.e., mandated treatment, individual therapy for a parent, protective services, juvenile justice programs).

As discussed previously, we suggest tailoring the content of the therapy from the FMC, beginning with clarification of realistic change goals, using incentives to promote positive behavior, improving monitoring, emphasizing SANE approaches to setting limits, problem solving, and negotiation. In family therapy, the number of sessions dedicated to each topic is determined by the family's adaptation of material. Issues of family context are addressed simultaneously with family management, continually empowering the adults in the leadership role in the family. Figure 6.3. provides an overview of the behavior-change cycle. Note that in the beginning stages of the change process, it is the therapist who more often actively structures and guides the intervention. Close to termination, the parent becomes more active in the change process, setting the agenda and guiding the work in each session.

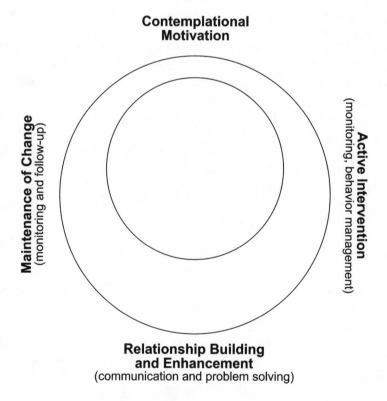

FIGURE 6.3. The behavior-change cycle.

SUMMARY

This chapter provides an overview of our menu approach to interventions supporting family management therapy. The FCU and a flexible intervention menu enhances the potential for initial engagement and shifting to more or less intensity in the intervention strategy, as needed. We address the delicate process of change by a variety of strategies. The first, training therapists to identify and work effectively with challenges to the change process, is critical.

7

Working with Adolescents

In this chapter, we provide an overview of our family-centered approach and discuss some process ideas in the context of a cognitive-behavioral approach to behavior change. It is often essential to complement interventions for parenting practices with those targeting the adolescent directly. A family-centered strategy for working with adolescents focuses on the goal of improving family functioning, and avoids interventions that directly or indirectly undermine parents.

RATIONALE

There are three major reasons why working directly with the adolescent is integral to the family-centered approach. First, to create change in families, it is usually necessary for the therapist to align and join with the "executive system." This can lead to adolescent alienation of the change process, which in turn can either increase conflict or reduce the likelihood of parental engagement. Often, parents take their cues from their teenagers concerning involvement in therapy. If an adolescent does not feel supported, she may encourage the parents not to get involved. Connecting and joining with the adolescent, in the long run, can often be in the best interest of the family.

If resources allow, finding the adolescent a separate therapist can communicate validation and provide advocacy for the adolescent in the change process (Chamberlain, 1994).

Second, by age 15, many adolescents are functionally autonomous. This means, simply, that there may not be an adult in their lives who is able or willing to take responsibility for guiding them. It is not unusual for parental illness or physical limitations to inhibit their presence in therapeutic activities. In such situations, the marginal involvement of adults can be used to support gains the adolescent makes in therapy.

Third, individualized work with an adolescent can benefit both the adolescent and family. From a life-course perspective, skills development and emotional well-being can be beneficial for both the adolescent, the current family, and possibly the next generation. We found that a cognitive-behavioral intervention with adolescents resulted in improved skills (Andrews, Soberman, & Dishion, 1995) and reduced coercive interactions between the adolescent and the parent in videotaped observation tasks (Dishion & Andrews, 1995).

Szapocznik and Williams (2000) reviewed evidence in favor of working with adolescents from a family-centered perspective, even when parents are unavailable for therapeutic involvement. Kazdin, Siegel, and Bass (1992) reported that interventions that target problem-solving skills, in addition to parent management training, are effective in reducing conduct problems in children. The important research of Lochman and colleagues (Lochman, Burch, Curry, & Lampron, 1984; Lochman & Wells, 1996; Lochman, White, Curry, & Rumer, 1992) clearly documents how a social-cognitive intervention for aggressive boys that includes goal setting reduced aggression in schools. Botvin and colleagues (Botvin, Baker, Dusenbury, Tortu, & Botvin, 1990; Botvin et al., 2000) effectively targeted life skills for adolescents to effectively prevent the emergence of drug use in early adolescence. Social skills training also has shown promise in reducing problem behavior in a variety of school and institutional settings (Bierman, 1990; Minkin et al., 1976). Both the science and our collective clinical experience suggest that the common underlying focus of successful interventions for adolescents is self-regulation.

We now discuss the developmental significance of self-regulation and the variety of strategies that promote self-regulation therapeutically.

A FOCUS ON SELF-REGULATION

Rationale

Developmental, neuroscience, and clinical researchers are converging on the concept of self-regulation as central to social and emotional adaptation and maturation. In particular, effortful attention control is a fundamental dimension of children's early adaptation pattern and is highly relevant to adjustment in childhood and adolescence (Kochanska, 1993; Rothbart & Bates, 1998). The voluntary control of behavior underlies the development of competence, reduced psychopathology, and physical health throughout the lifespan (see Figure 7.1). Bandura (1997) refers to this ability as "agency." Others refer to it as "emotion regulation" (Izard & Harris, 1995) and "executive functioning" (Barkley et al., 2001). Although researchers vary in emphasis and labels, it is safe to assume that most are interested in the ability to engage (or disengage) attention and behavior according to a consciously determined goal.

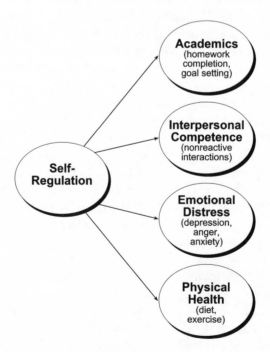

FIGURE 7.1. The development of competence, psychopathology, and physical health throughout the lifespan.

Although some self-regulation is certainly within the adolescents' temperament (Rothbart & Bates, 1998), the ability to regulate is learned through a variety of mechanisms, including classical conditioning (Rescorla, 1987), family interaction (Patterson, 1997), and peer environments (Dishion, 2000). Dynamic systems theorists discuss self-regulation as being embedded within self-organizing relationship systems (Fogel, 1996; Lewis, 2000).

The ability to regulate may ebb and flow with changing circumstances, corresponding to stress within an emotional climate (Izard & Harris, 1995). Simple changes in the brain, biochemistry, and cognition in adolescence are associated with relationship reorganization and temporary disruptions in self-regulatory abilities (Granic et al., 2003; Spear 2000a, 2000b). As shown in Figure 7.1, adolescent vulnerabilities in self-regulation may underlie the development of drug abuse (Dawes et al., 1999; Miller & Brown, 1991), problem behavior (Barkley et al., 2001; Barriga, 1997; Lochman et al., 1992), relationship satisfaction (Gottman & Levenson, 1986), stress and life management (Pulkinnen & Ronka, 1994), and physical health (Donovan, Jessor, & Costa, 1993).

Clinical Relevance

Even within conditions of stress, adolescent planning can protect youth in high-risk situations. Rutter (1989) describes research indicating that girls with a life plan are more likely to delay marriage and children for more favorable child-rearing circumstances, therefore improving their chances of positive adjustment after being raised in an orphanage. In an analysis of ATP data, Walsh (1999) found that girls who plan are less likely to be involved in a deviant peer group or to engage in precocious sex in adolescence. Conscious, effortful planning with realistic, attainable goals seems to be the foundation for coping with a variety of risk factors, for navigating adolescence, and for reducing the likelihood of substance abuse (Wills, Sandy, & Shinar, 1999; Wills, Vaccaro, & McNamara, 1995).

Effective cognitive-behavioral interventions target some aspect of self-regulation. Those that focus on emotional adjustment, such as depression (Lewinsohn & Clark, 1990), heavily emphasize monitoring emotions, making plans to engage in pleasant activities, and changing patterns of social interaction to improve satisfaction with relationships. Interventions that focus on adolescents with extreme levels of dysregulation, have more tools for supporting adolescent self-regulation, as exemplified in dialectical behavior therapy (Linehan, 1987).

INTERVENTION STRATEGIES

Our own intervention protocol with adolescents (summarized in Figure 7.2) is a curriculum called Teen Focus (Dishion, Moore, Prescott, & Kavanagh, 1989). Although it was designed for group interventions, it can also be used to support individualized work with an adolescent. As with most interventions that focus on self-regulation, we begin with a major emphasis on goal setting. Most young people have goals and are highly prosocial (Elliott & Voss, 1974). Unfortunately, those goals are often unrealistic. We work with adolescents to link their interests and current skills to define goals that they are likely to reach. Similar to our work with parents, we emphasize goals that are realistic, measurable, and under their control.

To attain goals and maintain motivation, adolescents often identify and seek support. Support is not a passive feature of the environment but, rather, is created by selection of individuals with consistent goals and contribution to a supportive relationship. We work with adolescents to identify friends, family, mentors, or other adults who might support their efforts to change.

The second major component of our intervention framework is

Goal Setting and Behavior Change
1. Achievable goals
2. Self-monitoring
3. Identifying supportive behavior
4. Reinforcement and motivation

Limit Setting and Self-Control
5. Making positive friendships
6. Controlling negative feelings
7. Setting limits with friends
8. Coping with adult limits

Maintaining Relationships
9. Listening and perspective taking
10. Bringing up a problem
11. Negotiation
12. Strengths and barriers

FIGURE 7.2. The Teen Focus curriculum.

to support setting limits on friends who may distract efforts to change, managing negative emotions, and coping with adult relationships. Finally, we develop interpersonal skills that will increase the adolescent's satisfaction with family and friendships. We include listening, perspective taking, negotiation, and problem solving in these skills.

The Teen Focus curriculum was designed to parallel that of the parent FMC. As discussed in Chapter 10, we discovered that aggregating the high-risk youth undermined the goals of the intervention and contributed to increases in some forms of problem behavior in the ATP adolescents. The focus of the curriculum, however, is of potential value when working with individual adolescents.

CHALLENGES IN WORKING WITH ADOLESCENTS

Despite the strong rationale for continuing to develop, refine, and articulate interventions that serve adolescents, there are challenges to working with adolescents from a family-centered perspective.

The Developmental Stage

Adolescents need increasing levels of autonomy, privacy, understanding, and validation from both parents and peers. Because of this dynamic, parents and adolescents may distance themselves from one another quite unconsciously (Steinberg, 1988). Changes in family structure (i.e., transitions) that coincidentally covary with puberty may have disastrous consequences. For example, a new stepparent or a new baby sibling during the adolescent phase can disrupt family relationships and in turn lead to escalation in a young person's problem behavior (Capaldi & Patterson, 1991). Under optimal circumstances, adolescence may be accompanied by conflict and increasing demands for independence (Granic et al., 2003). Under the worst of circumstances, it can lead to overinvolvement with peer groups that support problem behavior and maladaptive emotional coping (Dishion, 2000; Dishion, Capaldi, et al., 1999).

On the one hand, family-centered interventions can protect parents and teens from the vicissitudes of adolescence. On the other, therapy can amplify sensitivities and conflicts. For any individual, the therapeutic situation creates a sense of vulnerability. With adolescents, that vulnerability is magnified and includes not only the risks of disclosure and being misunderstood but also parental rejection, therapist evaluation, and loss of control.

As bad as things might be, teens typically have worked out some coercive or avoidance strategy to achieve their goals. The thought of having to change behaviors and ideas can feel frightening. Following from this, we find that the more we can make collaborators of adolescents at each stage of treatment, the more vulnerabilities are reduced and trust is built; also, the adolescents are less resistant to change.

Gender

Although parenting practices and behavioral expectations for boys and girls have become more similar during the past two decades, for the majority of teens, boys and girls have been socialized quite differently and present with different perspectives and concerns (Maccoby, 1992). We have found that it is important to consider gender as a significant variable in promoting adolescent engagement throughout treatment.

When we do workshops on treatment with adolescents and their families, we often hear about therapists' preferences for working with boys at this age. The discussion usually revolves around the perception that boys are less emotionally complex. There seems to be an underlying sense of a lack of control in working with adolescent girls:

"They just push and push, and won't quit."

"It's their mouths—they say the most cruel things."

"There can be so much emotion in the room, it takes the whole session to do damage control."

Girls often push against our implicit goals of keeping it brief and maintaining distance. We found that girls spend a good deal of time in treatment trying to create and then test their relationship with the therapist.

These processes can be understood within a socialization context (Maccoby, 1992). In comparison to boys, girls are typically socialized to display affiliative and affectionate behavior, which has been related to higher rates of affective disorders (Huston & Vangelisti, 1991; Kavanagh & Hops, 1994). Compared to boys, girls are typically socialized to be relationship oriented and, most specifically, oriented to the family. Following from this, problems are often best understood within a relationship context. We found that it is important to emphasize emotional regulation and clear boundary definition in the therapeutic relationship.

For boys, making the *process* relevant is often the biggest challenge. Work within a family-centered model will typically bring out issues of resistance to authority. The therapeutic relationship is often seen in terms of an interference with autonomy. From a socialization perspective, the family is a significant context in terms of a base of operations. From early in their development, boys are typically being pushed toward independent activities. Decision making outside the family and expression of aggressive behavior are normative.

There are many family situations that bring an adolescent to treatment. Although self-regulation can be seen as being "in the child," it can be addressed relative to family circumstances. Teens can discuss their goals with a parent, improve communication skills with adults, learn to accept limits from authority figures, make assertive requests, and seek support from well-meaning adults. These interventions are most effective when the therapist has successful engagement of the skills that are seen as serving the adolescent's interest.

ADOLESCENT ENGAGEMENT

The therapist strategies discussed in Chapter 6 also apply to work with adolescents. To develop a therapeutic alliance with an adolescent, it is critical to establish a collaborative set, to have a shared perspective, to be flexible, to be sensitive, and to work with their strengths rather than focus on weaknesses.

In addition to the common, nonspecific factors that are conducive to supporting change, work with adolescents requires additional skill. Therapists can make two common mistakes when working with adolescents. The first is to assume the role of "peer." This can be an effective short-term strategy for engagement, but it will eventually undermine the therapeutic relationship. The therapist working with an adolescent must assume the adult perspective solidly, while being sensitive to the unique awkwardness and complexity of adolescent life. The adult therapist does not explicitly or implicitly endorse anti-social attitudes, substance use, or other problem behavior by laugh-ter, attention, interest, or other reactions. The job of joining with an adolescent can require more clinical skill than when joining with an adult, because confrontation or advice may be perceived by the ado-lescent as unsympathetic, which disengages the youth from therapy. In the long run, it is better to connect with an adolescent as an adult rather than to connect by becoming a peer.

One solution to this dilemma is to become an advocate for the adolescent, especially when he and his family are participating in family therapy. By understanding the adolescent's perspective, you represent the adolescent in the family system. You have something to offer and can use that alliance to support and empower the adoles-cent's maturation and skill development in representing himself. Chamberlain (1994) describes the role of the youth therapist as the advocate in treatment foster care.

A pitfall of the advocacy model is the second barrier in working with adolescents. Often, youth therapists assume the adolescent's perspective and begin blaming the parent. Adolescents are quick to sense collusion on the part of the therapist against the parent. At times, it becomes necessary to take a unilateral perspective in physi-cally and sexually abusive families. Often, however, the antagonistic perspective of the youth therapist against the parents further weak-ens the potential for the parents to give care and guidance to their youngster. The therapist can best serve adolescents by empathizing with their perspective and tactfully reflecting the adult point of view. Role plays can be a fun way to assume the parents' perspective and allow the adolescent the emotional freedom to respond to parental behaviors in a way that promotes growth and development.

Figure 7.3 provides a pyramid model for guiding a therapeutic activity with an adolescent. The first layer of the pyramid is building a relationship of trust. As Carl Rogers (1957) pointed out years ago, the best way to build a positive therapist–adolescent relationship is to be genuine. This means be yourself—an adult providing support to a young person. Building trust and a positive relationship may take time, and it may require some activities that seem unrelated to therapy.

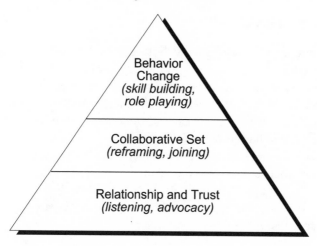

FIGURE 7.3. The therapy process pyramid in working with adolescents.

SOMEBODY IS WATCHING ME

Jack was 15 when he had his first psychotic break, with para-noid delusions. He was sure that his 14-year-old sister was col-luding with Satan to hurt him and their family. During an argu-ment, he became upset and attempted to stab his sister, who immediately ran for safety.

Jack spent the next year in the state hospital and became stabilized on medication. He was released to a treatment foster care setting, where one member of the therapeutic team sup-ported the foster parents, and the other attempted to build a trusting relationship with Jack. This meant weekly meetings playing cards, going for walks, playing video games, and simply talking. It took about 6 months to lay the groundwork, but when Jack's paranoid thoughts reemerged, he shared them with his therapist. Remedial action and support were provided for both Jack and his foster parents before the delusions were en-acted in the foster family.

A serious example such as this underscores the point that individual-ized interventions with adolescents are helpful for a wide range of cases. To establish therapeutic connection and maintain the family-centered emphasis, we recommend the following specific skills.

Explain the Process

Adolescents need to understand both their relationship to the therapist and what is expected in the therapy process. This begins in the initial interview and is an ongoing part of treatment. In the context of the advocacy role, it is best to define a therapeutic relationship as benefiting the family. This is easiest, of course, when parents are also engaged in the change process.

To counter feelings of vulnerability and divided loyalties, a definition that focuses on working with the whole family is best. Foreshadowing feelings that will likely occur, then checking in on the presence of these feelings throughout treatment, creates a respectful tone that teens appreciate.

> "As you may remember from our first meeting, what is usually helpful to teens and families is for me to help you express your point of view and to consider your parents, so that you and your family understand each other. There may be times when it will be important that we meet alone for this to be most helpful. Other times, you may feel like what's going on is unfair to you. I'm counting on you to let your family and me know that."

Predict Feelings

Even given this sort of explanation, it is not unusual, if you work individually with teens, for them to feel that you are "theirs," and to see any presentation of parental ideas or feelings as a betrayal. Many adolescents have experienced an association between disagreement and the end of a relationship. It is important to predict these feelings and concerns.

> "Because we're working together closely, we'll disagree sometimes. You may get upset, if it seems like I don't share your view. That's OK; we can expect that. It tells me that you're working on change and care about what happens when we're talking. Usually, when you get mad, it'll be because you think I just don't get what's going on. Our situation is an opportunity to talk about feelings safely. We'll talk about our disagreements and then continue."

Collaborative Set

The second stage in the change process is establishing a collaborative set. Integrating the work on motivational interviewing, this involves understanding where the adolescent falls in the stages-of-change continuum (Prochaska & DiClemente, 1982). This can be summarized and reflected from a variety of verbal and nonverbal behaviors. When the relationship is established, it is more likely that therapist efforts to articulate the adolescent's interests and concerns will result in a meaningful therapeutic interaction.

I JUST WANT A JOB

Matthew, a 16-year-old European American–American Indian youth, was abused by his parents and the system. At 6'1", he weighed about 240 pounds and had an anger problem. Upon his release from community detention, Matthew went into treatment foster care.

Because of his extensive history of both physical and sexual abuse, Matthew had difficulties establishing a trusting relationship with his therapist. His problem behavior would often escalate immediately following counseling sessions. From the therapist's point of view, these sessions were relatively benign. After a few disruptive outbursts, with relatively benign reactions from the therapist, Matthew began to engage.

One day, when discussing some difficulties he was having with his foster parents, Matthew blurted out, "I just want a job!" This was the third time he had mentioned work, so the therapist pursued this line of inquiry. Matthew was tired of being a child—he was ready to be treated like the man he physically appeared to be.

Given Matthew's intellectual functioning and academic history, he was unlikely to be acknowledged as a young man in the school setting. It became clear that counseling would be most successful if framed as "job training." The therapist and Matthew listed some basic skills that he would need to get and maintain a job (grooming, accepting feedback peacefully, talking, asking questions, staying calm). The foster parents then provided weekly ratings of these "skills," and in 6 months, Matthew was ready for his first apprenticeship janitor position.

Follow Their Lead

You can lead a horse to water but you can't make him drink. However, you can usually accomplish your goals by following an adolescent's lead to learn more about his perspective. Although, as therapists, we are all trained to be good listeners, this is an especially important skill in working with an adolescent. We often move faster than adolescents are ready to move, then become frustrated at their resistance.

At times it can be difficult to avoid thinking that the teen does not know what he wants. More often, this is an issue of trust: Therapists are adults, and other adults may have violated the teen's trust. We have found low-key sessions that serve to build a relationship with the teen is time well spent, listening and allowing the teen to size you up. Following his lead ensures that the therapist will offer a first step he can trust.

The Stress–Support Frame

Stress and support are words to which most adolescents easily relate, and they are useful in framing the issues brought to treatment. The importance of having support in life is made explicitly, along with identifying possible sources of support. Within a family-centered model, adolescents are guided toward gathering support from parents. However, for teens with many problems, it is often from peers that they can get unconditional support. Whether or not this is positive, it feels good, but until work is done on making choices from a place of self-care, it is not a good initial goal.

Sometimes a central goal of treatment is helping both teen and parent believe that the parent can be a source of support. A part of this process is helping to make teens' needs clear to the parents. Otherwise, such needs may be expressed through negative behaviors.

NOTHING BUT CONTEMPT

A history of aggressive behaviors, defiance, and disrespect toward his mother masked Marcus's need for parental support and attention. He was a 13-year-old middle child of an African American dad and European American mom. Marcus's withdrawn younger brother was the focus of his aggression, and his older sister, who was school phobic, received her share of Marcus's insults.

With Dad in jail, Mom was overwhelmed in dealing with the problems of the other two children and couldn't understand why Marcus was being so disrespectful. Because the therapist asked Marcus to discuss his stress and not his disrespect or co-operation with the family, Marcus felt understood and was able to begin expressing his needs.

Deciding to meet with Marcus alone eventually allowed the therapist to present Marcus's stress over the lack of any family support as the issue driving his negative behavior. This frame helped his mom develop some understanding and compassion for her son's expression of needs. This individual work was the first step on the long road to being able to work with Marcus and to help him and his mom see the possibility of her being able to offer support toward positive goals for Marcus.

Promote Self-Encouragement

An adult can reframe seemingly negative behaviors with positive motives. Robins et al. (1996) found that a positive reframe of adolescent behavior in family therapy increases the adolescent's constructive engagement in therapy and promotes a collaborative set within family therapy. Once behaviors such as *argumentative* are transformed into *invested*, *concerned*, or *caring*, a transformation takes place.

Adolescents often hear the negative message. Because of this, the positive countermessage may be enough to support behaviors that are consonant with the positive motivations. The therapist wants to promote the adolescent's recognition of his positive motivation and behavior, rather than being susceptible to adult definition. An important life skill is to learn how to provide self-encouragement. We begin this process early and explicitly by reflecting the positive efforts of the teen through our eyes, then giving assignments of self-recognition between sessions.

TECHNIQUES FOR BEHAVIOR CHANGE

The therapist–adolescent relationship and the collaborative set establish a foundation for behavior change. As discussed in previous chapters, a major part of behavior change is supporting motivation. Adolescents may not always agree with the vision of adults about what change is prioritized. On the other hand, if the information is presented in the right way, adolescents can make choices that are in their best interest. It is critical that the therapist provide "just enough" support and avoid undermining an adolescent's active effort to develop judgment and self-control.

Effectiveness in behavior change is enhanced by contextualizing the intervention. This means orchestrating environments that identify and support the behavior change. As structural family therapists have often told us, many problem behaviors emerge as a direct reaction to an intense emotional dynamic within the family. It can be enough to conduct systemic interventions that reduce the emotional valence of behavior change. For example, when parents in conflict communicate through the adolescent, the situation is best addressed by changing the communication patterns. However, in the face of barriers to parent change, the therapist could focus on separating the adolescent to extricate himself from this dynamic.

I WON'T TALK

Christian was being admitted to inpatient psychiatry by his parents at age 36. Although he was chronologically an adult, he remained functionally an adolescent.

Christian had difficulties beginning at age 17, when his brother committed suicide. One evening, Christian was talking about his brother at dinner with his alcoholic father and mother, when his father shouted, "Shut up!"

Christian did not speak again for 15 years. He was being admitted because his parents had finally given up trying to change his elective mutism, and because in the recent 6 months, he had shown signs of further psychiatric deterioration.

The moment Christian was admitted to the inpatient unit, several staff members told him that he would soon be talking. Staff and his parents alike attempted to force Christian to talk and eat. In providing consultation to the inpatient unit, we decided to use a paradoxical intervention to reduce the intensity around Christian's behavior change. In fact, when interacting with Christian, it was apparent that he had learned to communicate quite effectively, without actually talking. We constructed a contract with him to "not talk" during the next week. If he wanted to talk, he should choose a staffperson to whom he liked to speak, and he was to whisper only one word. He would earn a magazine if he chose to talk. The contract was shared with the nursing staff during rounds.

The next week, Christian fulfilled his contract. He spoke only one word to a staffperson of his choosing. We met and changed the contract slightly. He was only to speak two words. He agreed with this plan, the contract was signed, and it was communicated to the psychiatry staff.

Two hours later, we received a telephone call that Christian was talking. In fact, he had been talking for 45 minutes in milieu therapy—nonstop. This was the end of his 15 years of silence.

Paradoxical interventions can be useful to decompress the emotional intensity of the behavior-change process, not only for the adolescent but also for the surrounding environment. Prescribing the symptom, however, should only involve problem behaviors that are relatively benign (i.e., not harmful). Elective mutism is such a behavior. Note that behavior change in this case was initiated through changing the environmental reactions, not changing the adolescent. You might well imagine, however, that there was still considerable individual work to do with both Christian and his parents to support his independent living, to promote his use of constructive problem solving, and to help heal the traumatic loss of his brother.

When working with adolescents in support of behavior change, it is useful to collaborate with adults at home or at school. However, even with adult coordination, the best of plans can be undermined if adolescents are not fully involved in the change process. They also must understand that their self-interest is the central concern of the adults involved. Certain skills can be helpful in initiating and maintaining a behavior change plan.

Flexible Meetings

The major life issues with which teens struggle occur in the contexts of family and peer group. As anyone who has worked with adolescents knows, they are less comfortable than adults with a traditional approach to therapy (e.g., a 50-minute, face-to-face meeting with a therapist). We found that providing opportunities for interaction in a variety of settings promotes greater engagement and moves the treatment process forward. Individual therapy with an adolescent can occur in an office, a park, at a restaurant, or walking along the river or down the street. An added advantage is to work within schools, which affords the opportunity to include peers in meetings around problem solving and mutual goal development.

Working outside of the therapy room is also relaxing, which helps participation and frank discussion. Note that when the goal is to reduce adolescent problem behavior, and the therapeutic relationship is one means of engagement and support of improved family functioning, the interpersonal dynamic between the therapist and adolescent is less critical.

Giving Advice

For beginning therapists, for the sake of a therapeutic relationship, it is easy to hold off on giving advice to teens. However, expert advice is an important part of the therapist's role, and adolescents are there to hear that advice. It is rare to hear this from adolescents, but when it occurs, the therapist realizes the importance of their expertise.

When the question, "What do you think is important for helping people your age?" was posed to a 14-year-old African American boy in treatment for issues around his parents' divorce, he responded, "The advice about drugs."

> "But you've heard that before in school and from your family, haven't you?"
> "Yes, but I need to keep hearing it and thinking about it, so it will get in my head. And I respect you for telling me."

Research on therapist–adolescent interactions that promote behavior change (Chamberlain et al., 1984; Patterson & Forgatch, 1985) suggests that we use advice sparingly. Advice is especially useful in response to a question, coupled with a supportive relationship.

Objectification

Similar to our work with parents, we give adolescents the information we have about making changes. In this way, adolescents are full participants, with no hidden agendas. Although adolescents are brought to treatment by parents or other adults, the referral issues are not a mystery.

> "Your parents are concerned about your school behavior and the time you spend with friends. There's some information we've learned in working with lots of people your age that I think would be important to look at. Let's go through some questions together and get your point of view about what is affecting your school work."

The next stage in the objectification process is to conduct a functional analysis: Through a discussion, what are the antecedents and consequences of the problem behaviors? Given a positive relationship and a collaborative set, adolescents can identify fully the circumstances surrounding their problem behavior.

There are two main functions to problem behavior—positive reinforcement and escape conditioning. The former refers to situations in which the positive experiences emanate from the adolescent's problem behavior (e.g., drug use and other behaviors, organized partying, and other activities). Escape conditioning, in contrast, refers to behaviors that reduce or eliminate negative events. For example, not showing up to school can effectively eliminate the onerous task of attending high school and studying. This can be powerful in high school for young people who have a history of academic failure, especially when the discrepancy between their skills level and the academic demands is greatest.

> "So it seems that you have two things going on. By not showing up for school, you avoid dealing with Mr. Jones, your history teacher. Your sense is that he really doesn't like you. Not going to school also gives you time to hang out with your buddies. So there's a lot going on here. I can see why your parents are concerned, but I'm not sure why you'd want to change. Why would you want to change?"

Objectifying the adolescent's problem behavior and pointing out the pulls to continue with the same behavior is an excellent way to move into targeting behavior change that is meaningful to the adolescent, and identifying a strategy that addresses some of the dynamics that may serve as barriers to change. The functional analysis is really rather simple and should flow from a discussion of the events surrounding the problem behavior.

Tailoring Skills

Finally, to engage an adolescent successfully in a behavior change, it is necessary to tailor the focus to the adolescent's self-interest and current level of functioning.

I JUST WANT A JOB (CONTINUED)

"Okay, Matthew, our work together is going to focus on getting you ready to find a job. What skills do you think you need to improve for having a better chance at a job? (*Therapist and adolescent make a list on the board. The therapist suggests some skills and waits to get the adolescent's reaction before putting them on the board.*)

"This is a great list. There's one more skill I would like to suggest. In our work together, I've noticed that you're pretty sensitive to criticism. The pattern seems to be that when Bill (foster parent) corrects you, you really blow your lid. You get angry, and it's hard for you to calm down, right? Is this how you see it?

"Well, I'm here to tell you that you're going to work for people who will criticize you, and they'll fire you if you get really upset. I'd like to work with you on this. What I suggest we do is put down "Accepts Feedback" on your weekly card, so that we can talk about it and see if I can be helpful to you in this area. Getting good at accepting feedback will help you a lot when you get a job."

On the sensitive issue of accepting feedback, we were working with a young man who had an anger problem. Through the process described above, we were able to make progress in this area, in collaboration with the treatment foster care parents and school professionals. Eventually, the therapeutic relationship progressed to a point where the adolescent shared some of his thoughts and feelings when he was criticized. Given his extensive abuse history, his subjective experience during these times was emotionally intense. Working on relaxation skills and finding a context to discuss his horrible thoughts and feelings seemed to be the turning point. He no longer escalated out of control when confronted with a mistake.

Role Playing

Adolescents are dramatic enough that most will engage in role plays. Role play is skill building and helps the adolescent objectify his behavior in relationships. Humor is often appropriate. We always start off with "wrong-way" role plays: Asking the adolescent to demonstrate all the wrong ways of talking to a parent is a fun way to build discrimination training. After the wrong ways have been exhausted, it's time to try a positive strategy.

> "Okay, you be you and I'll be your parent. What should I say to make sure that you don't want to listen to me, or that the problem will not get solved (wrong-way role plays)? Now show me how I can bring this up so that your dad listens?"

This approach might be used to engage an adolescent who is shy or reluctant. Ascribing to her a role that is relatively easy to carry off ensures success and engagement in the role play process.

SUMMARY

Individual work with an adolescent is complementary to working with parents when a family-centered perspective is maintained. Adolescent therapy can be challenging because of the developmental and structural aspects of developing a therapeutic relationship. However, when developing a positive relationship, a collaborative set about the change process sets the stage for behavior change. Behavior change in the adolescent can influence the reactions and motivations of parents in a family-centered change strategy.

8

———

Working with Parents in Groups

Several of the best-practice prevention and intervention programs call for working with parents in groups. In this chapter, we discuss the advantages of working with parents in this way. In addition, we discuss some empirically based strategies for engaging parents in groups and managing group process to ensure the therapeutic goal of supporting family management.

RATIONALE

Many parents of adolescents prefer to meet in groups. Adolescence is a time of change and reorganization, often marked by increases in family conflict (Granic et al., 2003), in which parents find themselves challenged. Parenting practices that worked in the youth's childhood may be less effective in adolescence. New parenting skills such as negotiation and problem solving become more important. Parenting groups present an opportunity to share and hear the trials and tribulations of parenting adolescents, providing validation, support, and even inspiration.

In our original formulation of ATP, parent and adolescent psychoeducational groups were the central intervention strategy (Dishion et al., 1988). The work and success of Webster-Stratton and colleagues suggest that meeting with parents in groups, in conjunction with videotape modeling, can be quite effective in changing par-

126

enting practices (Webster-Stratton, 1990; Webster-Stratton & Herbert, 1993).

These outcomes applied to families of preschool children, but the findings also apply to work with families with substance-using adolescents (Friedman, 1989), except with perhaps higher rates of dropout (Lewis et al., 1990). Our experience over the past 15 years, and the intervention science literature, suggests the advantages and disadvantages for working with parents of adolescents in groups (see Figure 8.1 for a summary).

One of the most important advantages of group work is cost-effectiveness. One or two therapists with a group of 8 to 10 families can dramatically reduce the costs associated with typical parenting interventions. Parent group interventions that are guided by a well-established curriculum and parenting videotapes are more easily disseminated than family therapies, which may often require intensive training and supervision to establish independent competence. Parent groups are potentially more engaging compared to family therapy. The label "parent groups" reduces the stigma associated with traditional mental health services.

Working with parents in groups also provides therapeutic advantages to individual families. Most noteworthy is the social support function of group work. Social support can be especially powerful when parents are isolated, depressed, or undergoing transitions such as divorce or remarriage. In well-run parent groups, social sup-

Advantages	Disadvantages
+ Less stigmatizing	– Difficult to individualize
+ Social support	– Disruptive behavior
+ More discussion of norms	– Some parents may slip through the cracks
+ Group reinforcement	
+ Expertise opportunities	– 12 sessions, too few or too many?
+ Cost-effective	– More difficult to deal with emotions
+ Easily disseminated	– Higher dropout rate

FIGURE 8.1. The advantages and disadvantages of working with parents in groups.

port can turn into reinforcement for positive changes. For example, when a parent reports a success to the group, and the group responds positively, the reinforcement is often more powerful for maintaining effort than is a positive reaction from a therapist.

THE NEWLYWEDS

Reuben and Blanca married recently and were blessed with an instant family. From a previous marriage, Blanca had two adolescent girls, ages 13 and 14. Reuben, who had never been married, had no children of his own.

As often happens in stepfather families, Reuben assumed that it was his role to be a father to these young ladies, setting limits and intervening on an "as needed" basis. The effect was a disaster after only 3 months of marriage, and the bickering between the girls seemed to escalate.

The couple attended group regularly and worked on home practice. It was a matter of luck that there were two other stepfamilies in the group (one other couple had also married recently). This group constitution made it easy for the group leader to discuss frequently the special issues of stepparents, and to recommend a more "laid back" role for the new stepparents.

One week, during the setting-limits topic, Reuben and Blanca agreed to put both girls in a brief time-out when they argued excessively. There would be no more detective work to determine who was at fault. Blanca was the one to inform the girls about the change in plans and to set the limit, if necessary.

The intervention worked like a charm, and the couple was well on the way to working as a team and improving family relationships. Recounting this success to the group elicited a series of "oohs" and "ahs" from other parents, helping to consolidate the learning experience.

Group work with parents can provide a context for eliciting parental expertise that is not reflected in the curriculum. From an ecological perspective on parenting, there are many successful styles of parenting that cannot be fully addressed in any structured curriculum. Parents who share a cultural perspective can often provide wonderful ideas, strategies, or community resources that are helpful in managing family life and adolescents. Simply bearing witness to another family's success can prompt others' efforts.

A unique therapeutic advantage of group work with parents is the potential power of the group in establishing healthy norms for family management. We find this especially helpful for the meetings on setting limits, in which we structure discussions to actively discourage harsh or punitive parenting (see SANE guidelines in Chapter 6). Often, it is difficult for an individual therapist to address parental norms, but parent groups can be powerful in this respect. As discussed later, however, structuring discussions that lead to the establishment of healthy parenting norms requires leadership skills and professional training. Videotapes of positive and effective parenting are helpful for establishing a parent group atmosphere that supports and values family management practices.

Additional advantages also exist when conducting parent groups in school settings. For many families, schools are conveniently located. When conducting a parent group in a school, it is relatively easy to integrate school issues into the parenting discussion. We have found that it works well if school staff can be present during the first 30 minutes of the group. In the past, we have had school staff present the students' ABC (attendance, behavior, completion of school work) school monitoring report to their respective parents, and include data on attendance, behavior, and completion of homework.

Some disadvantages also exist when focusing on family management in groups. As suggested earlier, the group process can be difficult at times: Some parents may grab floor time, inhibiting other parents' opportunity to talk. Also, it is difficult to address individual concerns of families, especially when there is intense emotion in the room (e.g., a family undergoing divorce, a serious parental illness). During the course of a group, for example, it may become clear that some aspect of the discussion inadvertently has offended a parent. If the parent leaves before an opportunity occurs to discuss a concern, it may be difficult to keep her engaged. Parents drop out of individual family therapy, but it seems that they are even more likely to drop out of parent groups (Lewis et al., 1990).

Despite these disadvantages (see Figure 8.1 for summary), we recommend group work with parents when possible. In general, the advantages of group work outweigh the disadvantages. In the sections that follow, we have two levels of recommendations that help reduce the problems associated with group work. First, we provide an overview of the flow of the group with respect to content. Second, we discuss basic strategies for structuring groups to maximize the potential benefit to all group members. Finally, we discuss strategies for addressing common group process problems that may occur when running a parent group.

SESSION CONTENT

The FMC provides detailed suggestions on how to conduct a 12-session parent group with a family management focus, including exercises, rationales, role plays, forms, and an accompanying parent workbook for each session. An overview of the curriculum is provided in Figure 8.2. As discussed previously, the FMC also serves as a template for individual work with families, including brief, focused interventions and more extended individual family therapy with a family management focus.

There are three broad foci in the FMC: (1) using incentives to promote positive behavior change, (2) limit setting and monitoring, and (3) relationship skills, such as family communication and problem solving. The first phase of the FMC is the use of positive reinforcement programs to increase specific behaviors, such as cooperating with parental requests or doing homework. Well-used incentives can have a dramatic affect on reducing problem behavior and result

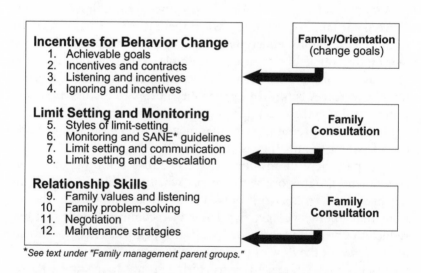

FIGURE 8.2. Outline for the Family Management Curriculum.

in a more positive family atmosphere. They are also the first step in supporting the parents as leaders in the behavior-change process.

The second aspect of the FMC is working with parents on setting limits and monitoring and on the articulation of rules (e.g., coming directly home after school, avoiding unsupervised homes). Limits are useless unless parents are willing to follow through with consequences. We promote the SANE guidelines for providing consequences. Discussion of these guidelines is a useful structure for helping parents evaluate their approach to limits and discipline.

The last but most important component of the FMC is relationship skills, which include basic communication skills (e.g., listening), problem solving, and negotiation. We address relationship skills last to avoid regressing into more conflict in families already struggling with family management issues. Relationship skills are not as useful when the source of conflict (cooperating with parents, school failure, and so forth) is ongoing.

BASIC STRUCTURE

Format

In general, we recommend that 8 to 10 families be represented in a group. Our experience is that half the participants are single-parent families or include families in which only one parent can attend the group meetings.

We suggest that the groups implement the FMC with schools or a neighborhood community service center. A parent group every season is one strategy to promote continued engagement. An advantage of ongoing or seasonal groups is that they promote parents' assuming more of a leadership role in subsequent groups. We find that parent assistants are quite useful in developing good discussions. The data also clearly reveal that paraprofessional therapists can produce outcomes comparable to those of psychologists (Christensen & Jacobson, 1994). Parent consultants could eventually conduct the group meetings, with the FRC staff assuming a supportive role. Funding is always a problem, and use of parent consultants is certainly a cost-effective strategy for maintaining parenting resources within the school context.

Consistent with research by Spoth and Redmond (1993), we suggest that the parent groups be offered on weeknights. In addition, parents prefer that the program be research-based and led by child development experts. We advertise the parent groups as the Adolescent Transitions Program (ATP) and describe it as a research-based parent group designed to help parents promote success in the adolescent years.

The FMC involves 12 sessions, with possible monthly follow-up meetings (Dishion et al., 2003). We suggest that the parent groups be led by a professional trained in mental health services, in general, and in leading semistructured groups, in particular. With the appropriate training, however, we suspect that paraprofessionals can be effective group leaders.

Attendance

Dropout is an added risk in parent groups. Our experience is that most of the dropout occurs *before* the first session. Dropout is also characteristic of substance-using families. It can be reduced, however, by therapists making visits to the home to engage parents (Szapocznik et al., 1988). In our first ATP parent group, approximately 30% of the parents attended. After a home visit, attendance increased to 70–80%.

A variety of strategies are useful for maintaining attendance. When parent groups are supportive, it is difficult for parents to stay away. Another strategy that many group leaders use is to share food during the meetings—perhaps potluck dinners, snacks, drinks (nonalcoholic), or other treats. Telephone calls between sessions can help prompt parents to complete the home practice, proactively problem-solve difficulties with the group, and maintain a personal relationship with parents. Brief consultations with families during the 12 weeks also help to maintain a personal connection and to tailor the curriculum to the needs of every family.

Parental involvement in the meeting agenda is a healthy strategy for promoting engagement. It may be useful to let parental interests guide the delivery of the content for the first four meetings, based on the FMC, then renegotiate at the end of that period. No data suggest that any aspect of this curriculum is superior; many families make changes at or after the fourth session.

We suggest regular (at least four) brief consultations with participating families to ensure that the material in the groups is addressing the weekly issues they confront in parenting. When resources are limited, a telephone call may suffice. However, it is preferable to meet with the family in person, in their home, in the FRC, or in some other community location that protects confidentiality.

Seating

Seating arrangements can help promote good group process and also be a tool to eliminate problems. Remember that the physical space can be altered. Change the seating arrangements to minimize conflict and to optimize collaborative interactions with parents. A semicircle is an excellent configuration, with the group leader and video player at the center. Groups also work well seated around a table, in a big circle, or even at individual students' desks.

As discussed in the FMC, the groups can be run effectively with one group leader; however, two leaders are optimal. Having a parent consultant is a cost-effective strategy for increasing the number of leaders in the group, although two professionally trained leaders improve the potential of the leadership team to identify and solve problems that emerge in the group process. When two group leaders are present, it is helpful to have them seated on opposite sides of the group, so that each has a unique vantage point. This also allows the two leaders to make eye contact easily and facilitates nonverbal communication. Coordination between the leaders addresses the needs of parents in the group with sensitivity.

Pacing

The pace of the content presented at each group meeting is an important strategy for maintaining engagement and promoting change. Leading groups teaches the importance of pacing content to the needs of parents in the groups, not to the needs of the group leader. The sessions have been designed to provide some flexibility with respect to the amount of material covered each time. It is vital that the group leader balance the pace with opportunities for parents to discuss their lives. Listing the agenda for each meeting on a white board or an easel sheet is a good way to earn the parents' permission to move ahead if the discussion gets bogged down. In addition, we have review sessions at the beginning of each meeting to ensure that all parents have an opportunity to talk about events in their family that occurred over the previous week.

Telephone Calls

An important part of parent support during the 12 weeks is midweek phone calls, which should be brief (5–10 minutes) and focus on checking on home practice and information covered in the meeting. You are calling to see if anything needs to be clarified and to find out how the parents' week is going. Parents often bring up issues that may be interfering with or supporting their parenting, which can help you in your work together in the group. One caution: Avoid making people feel like you are checking to see if the homework has been completed.

In 15 years of making telephone calls to parents, our experience is that, although it may take a few tries to reach them, parents are appreciative and in fact look forward to the calls. We also have found the calls to be great opportunities for individual support and recognition for parenting efforts in the midst of busy and stressful lives.

Humor

Parents will look forward to parent groups where appropriate humor is used to lighten the discussion and to increase the connection among group members. Humor can reduce the anxiety that some parents feel. Coming to each meeting should be a positive and even fun experience. However, we offer another caution: Overuse of humor can convey disrespect. Learn first how group members react to humor. To check reactions, we typically use humor about something we have personally said or done. This is an especially good idea in culturally diverse groups, where what may be humorous to one person can be something quite different for another.

Home Practice

The FMC is accompanied by a Leaders' Guide, which provides specific suggestions on running the parent groups. Each meeting has a home-practice component. Group leaders may encourage parents to engage in the home practice but *must* be cautious in communicating that a parent has failed if the home practice exercises were not completed. Any implication of failure may discourage attendance and reduce the likelihood of long-term change.

MANAGING GROUP PROCESS

Promoting Change

Unfortunately, many of our assumptions and guidelines for professional practice in providing mental health services remain unexamined by science (Dishion & Stormshak, in press). Much worse, several myths seem to be recalcitrant to change, even in the face of science (Dawes, 1994). We have no wish to perpetuate this cloud of misinformation on professional practice. Instead, we offer guidelines for managing group process that are strongly anchored in pragmatics of clinical experience, as well as in our own research on group interactions that predict change in parenting practices.

In our research, we videotape all our parent groups. We also ask parents and therapists to complete ratings of the meetings each week. We conduct these assessments so that we can examine which experiences in the parent groups predicted change and which were associated with parental satisfaction.

As usual, data have a way of revealing unfounded biases and assumptions. Our training in cognitive-behavioral therapy led us to a number of expectations that were not necessarily supported. The first was that the parent completion of home practice during the week would predict clinically significant change. The second was that therapist adherence to the written curriculum would be associated with home-practice completion and associated skills acquisition. Finally, we thought that family management skills acquisition would predict behavior change.

It is important to note that each of these constructs reflected individual differences among the parents in our original ATP study experiences in the parent groups. In general, we found little covariation between these constructs and changes in parenting behavior, as measured by comparing pre- and postobservations of parenting in a videotaped problem-solving task (Dishion & Kavanagh, 2002). In fact, contrary to expectation, we found that therapist on task was correlated negatively with change: The more the therapist rigidly adhered to the curriculum, the less the parent changed.

The picture was complicated by the presence of a bidirectional relation between parental behavior within the group and therapist reactions. It turns out that looking at clinically significant change clarified this confusion (Jacobsen & Truax, 1991). We grouped our families as deteriorated, improved, unchanged distress, and unchanged normal. When families were highly distressed at intake, therapists tended to be rated as more on task and effective by coders. We have come to call this the "emergency room" effect.

Analysis of the four groups described did suggest that positive group process differentiated the improved from the unchanged distress groups. A positive group atmosphere seems to account for the reduction of problems among those families in distress at intake (data are summarized in Figure 8.3).

More recently, Hogansen and Dishion (2001) reanalyzed the parent group data to understand the conditions under which parents were more likely to change. The videotapes of the parent sessions were recoded, focusing more on the various features of group process and based on the literature on effective group psychotherapy and motivational interviewing. Six constructs were measured, based on direct observations of each of the 12 sessions: therapist optimistic,

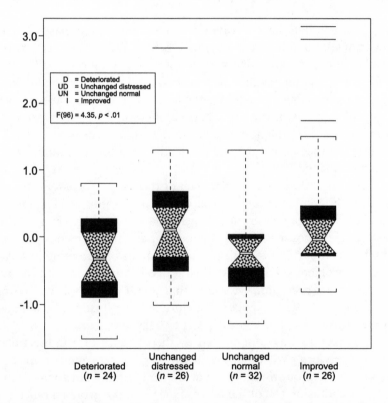

FIGURE 8.3. Observed positive group process and clinically significant change.

therapist reframe, therapist management of group talk, parent motivation, parent resistance, and parent group involvement. We analyzed the profiles of those families who made statistically reliable reductions in coercive interactions in their videotaped interactions with their adolescents. These data are summarized in Figure 8.4.

Although differences between those who changed and those who did not are discernible across all six constructs, only therapist reframe and therapist optimistic significantly differentiated the two groups. Therapist reframe describes a group leader's skill in taking parents' hopeless complaints and recasting them into statements that are conducive to change. For example, the therapist would respond to a parent's negative monologue about her adolescent son, Jerome, who she feels has a bad attitude about work, much like his recalcitrant and absent father.

BAD ATTITUDE

"Sounds like you've run into a wall with trying to get Jerome to help around the house. This is pretty common around his age. It may seem strange, but we may have to teach him how to be more cooperative. Let's see if what we talk about today is going to be helpful."

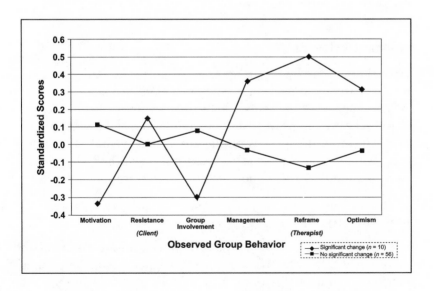

FIGURE 8.4. Profile analysis of behavior change in parent groups.

In this way, we help the parent move from an understandable place of hopelessness to one of putting in the work to make a family change. The implicit message is, "Jerome can change. He needs to be taught, like any child."

Embedded within the therapist reframe codes was an assumption of optimism about the change process. Therapist optimism was also a code in and of itself that differentiated between individuals who changed and those who did not. The group leader behavior that was coded as optimism was just that, the therapist's explicit tendency to be upbeat and positive about the prospect of making positive changes in families by focusing on family management.

An important note about this research is that the overall group effect on change in parenting was miniscule compared to the individual differences in how parents were treated in the groups. This is both a positive finding and one that suggests caution in how each parent is treated within a group. An overall positive group atmosphere will only carry part of the weight in behavior change; individualizing the intervention to each parent is also critical. Clearly, managing both aspects of the group (individual and group) requires more than a modicum of skill and clinical training. To this end, the following sections provide some suggestions on how to manage challenges to group process, with the goal of keeping individual parents engaged throughout the 12 sessions.

Personal Disclosure

Personal disclosure by the group leader is a delicate skill that should be used sparingly. If the leader is a parent, some acknowledgment of similar struggles or concerns adds to the group. In this sense, personal disclosure can provide support, validation, and a sense of optimism. However, the focus is on the group parents and their experiences. We find that parents learn best from each other's experiences. Parent assistants are also good resources for personal experiences.

Confidentiality

This is a common problem in groups of parents whose children go to school together, or who live in the same neighborhood. We establish a norm of confidentiality in the first session. The effect of the confidentiality norm seems to be that parents feel more cohesion and are more likely to attend to the concerns of other parents. We find that it helps to make this one of the guidelines.

Parent Recognition

We are living in a time of overscheduling for families. Parents may be juggling one or more jobs or going to school, along with parenting. If they are taking time to come to these meetings, their time in the group occurs in the midst of the rest of their already-busy lives. We acknowledge this each week by having a social or decompression time at the beginning of each meeting to help make the transition and get ready to focus on learning.

Parents come to parent groups with a lot of experience and have good information and support to offer each other. In all discussions, parents should be asked what they have been doing, and then be recognized for their efforts. Although this may seem like an obvious thing to do, we have observed that many leaders get carried away with presenting information and forget that this is not the first time parents have thought about or worked on these topics.

Asking parents what they are currently doing shows respect and gives the leader an opportunity to recognize positive practices. Often, parents use creative versions of the skills presented in the group that should be shared. We find that the more parental wisdom is incorporated, the more likely that parents will engage in the content. There is almost always something positive to pull out of just about any parenting example.

Parent Examples

As often as possible, refer to what parents have said and use their words to illustrate points in the curriculum:

> "Like Clyde said a few minutes ago, it can be hard to keep from getting upset. It's a great strategy to tell Sarah that he's feeling upset, and that he's going out on the porch for a few minutes before they talk any more."
> Or:
> "The story Annette just told about calling Jason's mom last weekend is an excellent example of following up on rules and networking."

Both are examples of the group leader linking parents' stories to the FMC.

DIFFICULT SITUATIONS

A Parent Talker

Many parents have a lot to say and no willing audience. Coming to a parent group can provide this audience. One of the group guidelines we use is to share talking time. However, a parent commonly may attend a meeting where she needs to do a lot of talking, and ignore guidelines. Group members may begin to show restlessness or discomfort, and it can be a delicate balance to show respect for both the individual parent and the rest of the group. Usually, acknowledging the parent's situation and asking to continue the discussion after group moves things along and draws closure.

We have several strategies if this becomes a problem in more than one meeting. As a preventive step in the first group meeting, we say that we may need to interrupt parents from time to time to keep our commitment to the group as a whole to cover the material. This gives back control to the leader in the case of a talkative parent. Then, if this scenario occurs, the leader taking responsibility can say she has noticed that the group is falling behind in covering the information. This sets up a context for tabling the discussion.

Another strategy we use is to make an agenda with a time line for the meeting. Asking the "talker" to help keep track of whether topics are being covered in a timely way works well. Yet another tactic is talking to the parent outside of the group. Acknowledge that she has information to share, then ask if she would like to meet individually, since you do not want to take too much time away from other parents during group. Getting to this place is rare given that group process and other strategies usually take care of parents who have a lot to say.

"War" Stories

It is easy for parents to get involved in lively discussions of personal issues that may not be related to the meeting topic. Also, many parents are isolated in their parenting and do not have places for discussion. A common occurrence in groups of parents who struggle with challenging children or situations is the telling of "war" stories. These stories usually do not offer examples of positive parenting, but instead create a context of discouragement and hopelessness about change. Leader pacing and process guidelines can curtail these stories.

Older Children

Many parents will have older children, which can be a plus or a minus. If they have parented an older child successfully, then a child who is not responding in the same way (which is more common than not) can be confusing. Conversely, when parents have had problems with an older child, they will want to bring up past problems or ongoing difficulties with that child.

When parents are discouraged, they can bring a lot of negativity and helplessness to the group. We found that group members often intervene and give parents support to counter discouragement and negativity. We have heard more than one parent tell another, "Each child brings a parent something different" or "You can't live in the past." These times are also good opportunities for parent helpers to share their experiences with a difficult child.

When group members do not intervene, one thing that works well is to acknowledge feelings and frame group time as an opportunity to focus on one child, without the emotional overtones that occur at home. Also, if the youngest adolescent is the easier one, we typically suggest practicing with him, then applying the skills to the older sibling.

Extreme Stress

Parents often bring everyday stresses to group. Single parents can feel overwhelmed with little adult support at home, and couples often struggle with two jobs. It is good to allow some discussion and support from the therapist and the group, then frame the stress as something to work around, in order to stay on track with parenting. For example, feelings of depression can create barriers to spending time with teens, and to being positive and supportive.

Unfortunately, in the course of 12 weeks, a major life event may be brought to the group, such as an impending divorce, victimization, serious illness, or even a death in the family. All these events have happened in our group work, creating emotionally powerful moments.

It is important that parents share their burdens and for group members to be able to offer their support and acceptance. When sensitive information is being presented, ending the discussion can be delicate. We usually say that if people want to talk more, we can make time at the end of group.

Rarely in our experience have members not been able to turn back to the curriculum. If the stressed parent is able to come to group, she most likely can and wants to return to the lesson. After group, if it seems appropriate, asking the parent under stress if she would like an individual meeting or a referral offers good support.

Conflict

Even if you have group guidelines, conflicts can arise in any group of people. The struggles of parenting can touch people's hearts and souls. There can be a lot of strong beliefs and stories about why things are the way they are.

If you are conducting a parent group within an existing context such as a school or community center, the parents may know each other. Points of conflict can involve other families and children in the group. Parents or their children may have had conflicts in the neighborhood or at school. We have had more than one parent group in which one child is seen as "the bad kid" who is leading another child down the wrong path. We have also had other parent groups in which parents make a point of distancing themselves from another parent or grimacing at a parent's comments.

If conflict occurs between two parents, our first strategy is to ignore it, unless it is taking up group time or causing other group members distress. Once in a while, a conflict may interfere with the group. When that happens, talking to parents separately outside the parent group, acknowledging the conflict, and asking what they think they can do, so that both can stay in the group, puts the solution in their hands. If they are not sure, offer to dismiss the issue in an individual meeting to decide if the group will meet their needs. This solution usually works, because parents want to stay in the group. In our experience, we are not aware of any parents who have left the parent group because of a conflict with another parent.

If the conflict is between couples, we discuss their differences outside of the parent group and ask what they think they can do to work together during the meetings. We have had individual meetings to set up strategies that couples can use to avoid openly disagreeing during group.

WEATHERING THE STRUGGLE

Zena was the member of a group, along with six other families of seventh graders from the same middle school. She was originally the only single mother in the group and took a me-versus-them stance.

After several meetings, the health of one of the fathers took a serious turn, so, in essence, there were two single parents, which still did not diminish Zena's feelings of discrimination.

Zena also had an ongoing conflict with one of the couples in the group, related to some trouble in which their sons had been involved. Interestingly, Zena would usually sit next to these people in group, so that she could turn her back to them dramatically.

She also had a counterculture lifestyle, which she seemed to wear proudly, yet, conversely, she felt the need to explain it.

In her first individual family meeting, Zena self-described that she did not feel comfortable disciplining her kids, because it brought up all the abuse she had suffered as a child. During the group meeting on family rules and limit setting, an explosion occurred.

In a brainstorming activity on family rules, the leader queried Zena's response, which was meant to clarify Zena's rule structure. Zena took this as criticism and an indictment that she had no rules, so she lashed out at the leader, using several strong expletives. The group was noticeably shocked, and before the leader could respond and clarify, group members jumped in to ask why Zena was so upset. This allowed the misunderstanding to come out for clarification and also an opportunity for the group to support Zena and show that no one was judging her.

This uncomfortable outburst and the lack of censure that followed led Zena to apologize later to the leader and request help with her own insecurities as a parent. Zena's continuing work on trying to improve things in her home was recognized, and a suggestion was made that she seek individual counseling to work on issues around her previous abuse as a child and numerous sexual assaults as a teen and young woman.

SUMMARY

In this chapter, we have focused exclusively on working with parents of adolescents in groups. There are several advantages to group work with parents, which, in many circumstances, offset the disadvantages. We suggested the use of the FMC and outlined the basic format for the groups, strategies for managing the process in the group, and higher order skills for promoting change and constructively working with challenging situations.

PART IV

School and Community Change

Chapters 9, 10, and 11 are concerned with the issues of integrating a family-centered perspective within school and community systems. In Chapter 9, we discuss specific strategies for implanting ATP within public schools, addressing the varying dynamics of this particular service delivery system (Hoagwood & Koretz, 1996). Although schools may be a convenient access point from a public health perspective, lack of resources, training, and leadership can dramatically compromise efforts to engage parents and families.

In Chapter 10, we discuss the details of findings from the research on ATP over the past 15 years and provide the scientific justification for promoting parenting practices and avoiding aggregating youth into programs that may inadvertently do harm. The chapter reveals that working collaboratively with parents within a school system can reduce problem behavior and shows that our ATP strategy is realistic with respect to professional time and energy.

Finally, in Chapter 11, we discuss diverse strategies for evaluating family-centered interventions. We provide four useful evaluation strategies that can be used to establish a service through a granting mechanism, when justifying a family-centered intervention in other service delivery systems, or in evaluating policies promoting community change.

The link between Chapters 9, 10, and 11 is the concept that data and science are critical for change at all levels of analysis. For schools, having a well-organized system for labeling positive and problematic student behavior, and recording daily student behavior, provides a foundation for being effective with parents in schools. Monthly or weekly graphs of student behavior in schools can provide school professionals with the information needed to make good decisions about prioritizing energy and time.

Randomized intervention trials are one important tool for making critical decisions about what strategies are most likely to be effective, or perhaps more important, culling those interventions that might do harm. Collecting periodic data on families in treatment, on the effectiveness of services, or even on communities making change is the best strategy for ensuring a solid foundation of progress.

9

Family-Centered Intervention
in Schools

This chapter describes the components and activities of the FRC that can be used in a public middle or high school environment. The multilevel model described in Chapter 2 provides the organization of the FRC services. The therapist in the FRC assists in establishing a helping system for each student by promoting collaboration and consistency between the home and school. As discussed in Chapter 2, to have a public health impact within a neighborhood and school, it is necessary for the FRC therapist to deliver universal, selected, and indicated level interventions.

THE FRC AS A UNIVERSAL

Before going into details of the specifics of each component, we think it is important to discuss the methods and goals of universal prevention strategies. The Institute of Medicine (Mrazek & Haggerty, 1995) describes a universal preventive intervention as "targeted to the general public or a whole population group that has *not* been identified on the basis of individual risk. The intervention is desirable for everyone in that group" (p. 24). When thinking about the effectiveness of a universal intervention, we should consider a range of direct and indirect effects. For example, the parenting universal described in this chapter has a number of goals related to the reduction of problem behavior. Direct effects mobilize parents to use protective parenting strategies during their children's early adolescence to reduce risk for substance use and other problem behavior. Indirect effects include information dissemination regarding the FRC, parenting resources, and developing a culture within the school community that is supportive of parenting.

From a public health perspective, universal interventions are of major relevance to the reduction of problem behavior in children. When applied to an entire community, even a small effect size can be significant (Biglan, 1992). To realize this goal, universals must be relevant to the full range of parents, including those with strong parenting, and those with a history of poor parenting practices. The support of existing parenting efforts serves to strengthen the community against future family disruption.

To be effective, a universal intervention must facilitate a series of interactions within the adult world that directly and indirectly affect parenting practices. Figure 9.1 provides an overview of the cycle of community change facilitated by the FRC model. Classroom-based activities inform students, teachers, parents, and school staff of family and parenting issues. Proactive identification and parental engagement reduce risk of a student's problem behavior by mobilizing parenting and improving communication with school staff.

We have learned over the years to think and work ecologically to enhance the impact of the universal, shaping services to fit the needs, interests, circumstances, and resources of each school. Our model of the development of problem behavior and the family-centered approach allows us to prioritize the FRC therapist activities. For example, periodic telephone calls to parents about their teenager's behavior at school are likely to be more helpful in promoting success than is a large parent meeting on adolescent self-esteem. In fact, we find ourselves frequently engaged in a variety of brief interactions that facilitate communication with staff and parents.

DEVELOPING A TEAM

A major area to consider with parents who facilitate communication when establishing an FRC is the dynamics of working in a school. Despite the theoretical appeal of placing schools in the center of pre-

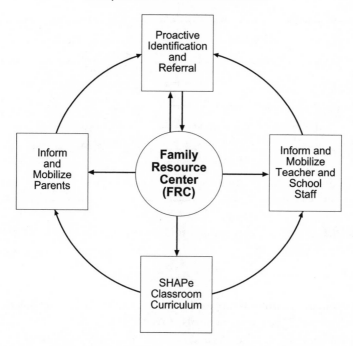

FIGURE 9.1. Cycle of community change facilitated by the Family Resource Center.

vention activities, there are also formidable barriers (Walker, Colvin, & Ramsey, 1995). Teachers, counselors, and principals are preoccupied with teaching, handling crises, and managing the day-to-day affairs of a typical middle or high school. It is not surprising, then, that a major factor in program acceptance and adherence is the extent to which the intervention requires *additional energy* from school staff (Walker et al., 1995).

It is important that school staff value the FRC activities, and that strong support come from the school leadership and teachers. Workshops, attendance, participation in major staff meetings, and flexibility are the ingredients necessary for a successful implantation of the FRC. Even under optimal conditions, it takes time for school staff to begin using the FRC in their response to student issues. Figure 9.2 shows the number of family contacts and referrals in the first 2 years of an FRC in a typical middle school.

A family-centered universal intervention that minimizes school

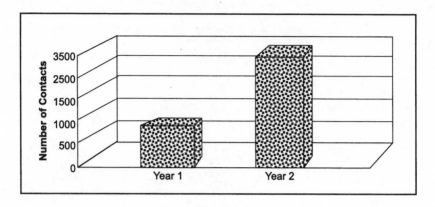

FIGURE 9.2. Number of parent contacts in the first 2 years of a Family Resource Center.

staff time and complements existing educational practices has the potential for acceptance by schools. Over the past 10 years, there has been an increase in the "full-service school" (Walker et al., 1995). Schools in inner-city settings typically provide breakfast and lunch. Health clinics are an important addition to schools, especially those that educate adolescents. The FRC is an excellent complement to these services within schools.

Most school professionals simply are not trained to work collaboratively with parents. In one district meeting we attended, 100% of the 15 participating middle school principals volunteered their schools for pilot testing of the family-centered interventions described in this volume. We believe that was because the intervention program targeted two major concerns of these school leaders: problem behavior and working with parents.

Bringing additional resources to overburdened schools is enormously helpful in program acceptance. However, there is a necessary integration process before an FRC becomes part of a typical school. A major principle of prevention science is integration of a universal intervention within existing service delivery systems (Hoagwood & Koretz, 1996). The process of integration is summarized by phases:

1. An informal discussion with the school community leadership (e.g., principal, counselors, parents, teachers), in which there is an exchange of information regarding existing services and the po-

tential for collaboration. Cultural diversity and resources within the school also need to be discussed and respected.

2. A meeting with the majority of school staff regarding the role of the FRC therapist, the classroom curriculum, and the kind of information and services available. It is important to provide confidentiality guidelines in advance of any family intervention, understand school policies, share counseling guidelines, and promote professional communication.

3. Implementation of the SHAPe (*Success*, *Health*, and *Peace*) curriculum in a health or homeroom class, with distribution of newsletters to parents, teachers, and other relevant school staff.

4. Media (e.g., public-access television) and focused family-centered presentations to parents, students, and school staff.

5. Orientation meetings for parents at the beginning of the school year, including self-assessment, needs identification, and proactive information regarding schoolwide discipline plans and policies.

6. Informational brochures on parenting and adolescent development.

7. Attendance at all major meetings involving teachers and parents, when activities or family work conducted through the FRC are discussed.

8. Informal daily interactions with teachers, principals, counselors, and parents that promote discussion of the parents' positive attributes and successes.

If these steps are completed within the school year, the school staff should have a reasonable understanding of the range of services, and the kinds of referrals and interventions that constructively involve parents. However, it takes time to develop a shared understanding about the value of taking the extra time and energy often required to incorporate parents into the school's operating system.

THE OPERATING SYSTEM

In the last decade, considerable progress has been made in working in school environments to reduce problem behavior by virtue of clarifying expectations and using well established, school-based interventions (Gottfredson 1988; Horner, Day, & Day, 1997; Sugai et al.,

1999). Unorganized, chaotic schools lead to parental disengagement, ineffective problem solving, unclear and biased identification of risk, apathy among staff, and higher rates of problem behavior. Promoting improved organizational functioning, especially around schoolwide behavior management practices, provides a foundation upon which parenting interventions are based. An effective behavior support strategy (Sugai et al., 1999) for improving the school operating system is an excellent foundation on which to build an FRC.

Central to improved organization is a referral and reporting system that is proactive and clear. For instance, many schools do not record discipline contacts or collect monthly data on referrals, and so forth. Standardizing and using software programs to manage referral data can motivate school change. Regular reports to school staff on trends in student success and difficulties can facilitate problem solving. Such an operating system is crucial to the goals of proactively identifying youth in the school system who are in trouble, engaging parents at the right time, and increasing motivation for parental maintenance of a positive behavior management plan. The interface between the school operating system and the role of the FRC is discussed below.

THE FAMILY RESOURCE CENTER

Activity in the FRC serves two functions. The first is a preventive function for families at little or marginal risk. The second is a gating function, which directs individual families to resources that are most palatable and appropriate to their level of need. Chapter 5 provides more detail on the FCU, the key intervention for families at risk either through self-identification or by referral from school staff.

The Setting

The development of an FRC provides the basic foundation for systemic change. The center can be both a physical and a psychological space for parents, similar to the teachers' lounge. It is a good idea to provide coffee and other amenities, if space and resources permit. Material resources needed to establish an FRC include the following:

1. An available room for confidential meetings with parents, students, and teachers.
2. Parenting- and family-centered literature of interest to a wide range of parents of diverse cultural traditions.
3. A variety of teen- and family-centered literature of interest to young adolescents.
4. Furniture that creates a warm, inviting atmosphere and is conducive to discussion.
5. A telephone for daily calls to families and an answering machine that provides general information for parents and allows them to leave messages.
6. A video camera for recording parent–child communication in family assessments, preferably one that can be taken to family homes.
7. A videotape player, television, and, optimally, earphones and a private viewing location.
8. A computer with software that enables the FRC staff to easily generate interesting newsletters and individualized reports to parents regarding their child's attendance, behavior, and completion of assignments.
9. A locking file cabinet to store family information.

Staffing

We refer to the primary professional staff as a "therapist" to distinguish the training and skills required to collaborate with parents. However, our FRC staff are master's-level clinicians; therefore, given the proper training, such a staff could be full-time school counselors. We estimate that one full-time counselor in the FRC can provide the range of services in a typical middle school environment. In culturally diverse schools, we recommend that the one position be divided among two or three staff members to represent the diversity of families in the school.

In training, we emphasize knowledge of empirically based parenting interventions, such as those provided in this volume, or those established and tested for parents with younger children (Webster-Stratton, 1990). One activity that promotes knowledge of effective parenting interventions is tailoring the content of the curricula into brochures and handouts for parents. In addition, a series of training sessions on working collaboratively with parents is essential. The basic principles of this work with parents are outlined in Chapter 6.

Informal Communication

It is important to take the time to understand existing communication systems, and high- and low-stress times of the day. It is also helpful to become acquainted with how problems are solved and identified. Unfortunately, because of the incredible demands on teachers and counselors to provide surrogate parenting, mental health services, and policing, the school staff are often handling a crisis. Although there were clear crisis situations, we found that the majority of problems did not reach this level of intensity, but were perceived as such because of time demands for resolution and limited staff resources. Despite accepting the school's position, the FRC consultant remains outside the response mode in order to be a more effective resource. When confronting problem behavior in the school setting, we first gather information and then develop strategies in collaboration with parents and school staff.

Proactive Neutrality

This is often the most difficult aspect of work between schools and parents. School staff and parents have preestablished opinions of one another, comprising an interesting mix of reality, gossip, and personal histories. These can be valid and accurate opinions, or they can be skewed.

Blame never solves problems; therefore, FRC staff must remain neutral. The therapist can be most helpful by taking a proactive stance to minimize future difficulties through a collaborative problem-solving model. Being proactive includes frequently interacting with school staff and planning to prevent anticipated problems or to reduce the reoccurrence of long-standing student difficulties. For example, violence within a school setting can often be anticipated by observing the patterns of peer interaction (i.e., teasing, rumors, challenging, and group interactions), which may provide an occasion for proactive planning with respect to a parent meeting on preventing violence. The FRC staff cannot afford to wait for problems to be delivered to their doorstep.

Establishing the FRC in a middle school is not sufficient as an overall prevention strategy. We have staffed FRCs and know that books can be written between meetings with parents in some schools. In fact, one elementary school we staffed did not provide one referral for the entire year. The use (or lack thereof) of the FRC is a systemic issue related to the activity, collaboration, and integration processes of the FRC staff. When principals, teachers, counselors, and other school colleagues are knowledgeable about the FRC services, more families in the population benefit. For this reason, we designed the classroom curriculum, which includes a series of parent–child exercises that involve parental input around themes relevant to family management practices.

ENGAGEMENT STRATEGIES

In-Class Curricula

Most public middle schools are inundated with classroom curricula to prevent violence, drug use, and unsafe sexual practices. There is considerable empirical support for school-based prevention curricula having a direct effect on young adolescent behavior. Most exemplary is the work of Botvin and colleagues (1990), whose curriculum focuses on resisting social influences to use drugs, emphasizing cognitive-behavioral change strategies.

It is an interesting sociological note that the majority of these prevention programs presume that serious behaviors can be prevented without engaging the cooperation of parents. It is quite possible that by creating polished, flashy, school-based curricula to prevent drug abuse, violence, and unsafe sexual practices, we inadvertently give parents the message that these issues are no longer their concern.

Early on in our experience with piloting the FRC model, we discovered that engaging parents requires leaving the FRC and going into the classroom. The main rationale for going into the classroom was to communicate important information about family management to parents through classroom activities. Moreover, a review of the literature reveals that prevention programs that incorporate homework assignments for parents show promising effects in the reduction of smoking (Telch, Killen, McAlister, Perry, &

Maccoby, 1982) and drug use (Pentz et al., 1989) in middle school and beyond.

FRC staff involvement in the implementation of the SHAPe curriculum serves three functions: (1) support for teachers conducting an empirically validated intervention in homeroom or health classes; (2) interaction with teachers and other school professionals around the theme of prevention, adolescent health, and parental involvement; and (3) building the parenting strengths and resources in the school community.

To mobilize parents in a school system, we need literally to reach out through classroom activities. However, to engage the majority of parents, we focus on current parenting strengths. Parent–child activities are designed to elicit competence and positive norms that promote adolescent success and well-being.

In the SHAPe curriculum, each of the 6 weeks includes a home exercise designed to motivate positive parenting practices. For example, on the topic of academic success and homework goals, we ask each family to report effective methods of encouraging homework, the amount of time spent reading and doing homework in an average school day, and what incentives are used to encourage homework. FRC staff summarize these reports in a brief newsletter that is sent to all parents of students in the classroom. If you work across grade levels, results can be summarized by grade, allowing parents to gain information on effective developmental changes in parenting practices. We share information about parenting practices related to academic success and learning that parents and teachers would not have otherwise. At the end of each SHAPe newsletter is the name and contact information for the FRC therapists. Materials and videotapes are available for parents who want more information on each curriculum topic covered.

Topics covered in the curriculum and the corresponding parent–child activities (Kavanagh, Dishion, Winter, & Burraston, 2000) include the following:

Week 1: School Success

Class lesson: Setting goals for school success, structuring time and places for doing homework, and the importance of incentives.

Family home activity: Discussing and sharing successes to encourage homework completion and use of incentives (positive reinforcement).

Week 2: Health Decisions

Class lesson: Defining healthy behavior; setting norms for diet, sleep, exercise, and drug use; and seeking the company of peers and adults who value health.

Family home activity: A communication exercise on drug-use norms and a stimulus to solve the problem of teen smoking (limit setting on drug use).

Week 3: Building Positive Peer Groups

Class lesson: Discriminating between healthy and unhealthy peer activities; identifying individual peer activities and friendship qualities that promote success, health, and well-being; and peer resistance skills.

Family home activity: Discussing and sharing information about parent strategies for limiting access to risky peer activities and community hot spots, and sharing opportunities for supervised activities after school (monitoring and relationship quality).

Week 4: The Cycle of Respect

Class lesson: Identifying the cycle of respect and discussing adult limit setting as risky situations for disrespect and conflict; and strategies for dealing with adult limit setting.

Family home activity: Discussing and sharing successful strategies to promote respect and handle disrespect in families (limit setting, coercion).

Week 5: Coping with Stress and Anger

Class lesson: Discussing warning signs of anger and strategies to handle anger constructively.

Family home activity: Discussing and sharing positive strategies for dealing with anger in the family (limit setting, coercion)

Week 6: Solving Problems Peacefully

Class lesson: Discussing a constructive approach to negotiate conflict, which involves three steps: bringing up the problem neutrally, checking out the other person's point of view, and listening skills.

Family home activity: Discussing and sharing family strategies to negotiate conflicts; having the family conduct a listening exercise (problem solving and listening).

Implementation Issues

This 6-week curriculum is meant to be an overview of skills and strategies. It is not designed as an intervention for serious behavioral or emotional problems. Consistent with the research by Botvin and colleagues (1990), we recommend using older, successful students to facilitate the discussion and model role plays. This needs to be arranged well in advance to allow high school students to sign up and earn credit for the activity. We also have recruited college students. They are still young enough to bridge the gap between early adolescence and adulthood and have credibility for both students and teachers.

We use group incentives both for participating in the class activities and for completing home activities with parents. Incentives may include grades for participation and food for class parties (i.e., pizza). Choice of incentives should be guided by class size, resources, and the number of students who are potential behavior problems. The specific recommendations for behavior management are found in the SHAPe leader's manual (Kavanagh, Dishion, et al., 2000).

When SHAPe is included within a middle school curriculum, one incentive is to base grades partially on completion of student homework activities. As with many assignments, students are expected to engage parents for 15 to 30 minutes per week on the weekly SHAPe topic, in order to pass that aspect of the health curriculum.

The curriculum requires 6 weeks to administer and can be carried out within one 40- to 60-minute class period. FRC staff typically lead the SHAPe classes; classroom teachers are also appropriate, if given some level of training and support by the FRC staff. What makes these classes well received is that they promote discussion and student activity. Peer counselors and parent volunteers can be helpful with the delivery and preparation of newsletters to family and school staff. We recommend that SHAPe classes be implemented in the early fall of each school year, in order to inform and engage parents early in the school year.

The SHAPe curriculum is a major activity of the FRC. Other strategies at the universal level are also important to the goal to support parenting of adolescents.

Use of Media

Parenting information can be delivered effectively with videotapes or other media. Public-access television can be used to provide direct modeling to parents who participate in the SHAPe class. Some public-access television stations have recording studios. Regardless, the FRC staff can videotape one family each week that engages in the home activity. The FRC staff, the principal, or even a student, can narrate the videotaped family activity. Successful students and families representative of each community should be selected for these media activities.

It is critical to have families representative of the cultural diversity of their community. Each week, then, families can turn on the television and watch a family from their community carry out the activities. Several different families can model each activity, or a set of families can rotate across the six activities. The SHAPe curriculum provides a framework of the skills to be presented each week. In addition, in completing the home practices activities, families contribute "local norms" about supervision, homework activities, and other parenting themes that can be communicated in newsletters at the end of the 6 weeks.

A central principle of prevention is community ownership of the ideas and strategies being promoted (Kelly, 1988). When entering a school system, it is essential to identify parents, teachers, or other community leaders, and to solicit their involvement and ideas. With individuals that represent strong leadership for youth abstinence and parental involvement, creative strategies can be used to collaborate in developing media that are relevant and salient within each community. The school orientation meeting and parent self-assessments can also be put on public-access television.

Orientation Meetings

Most schools have parent orientation meetings at the beginning of the school year; many of these are well-attended. The FRC staff should take an active role at these meetings to inform parents of the resources and goals of the FRC. Specific presentations can be made to parents about FRC and services for the year.

In addition, the FRC orientation with parents can involve a family self-assessment exercise. Self-assessment is integral to developing motivation to change. Parents view a videotape we developed, *Parenting in the Teenage Years* (Dishion, Kavanagh, & Christianson, 1995), that presents an array of adolescent problem behavior, and parent reactions are displayed to allow the parents to self-assess their own parenting practices. Parents complete a brief inventory while watching the videotape to indicate an interest in FRC resources at the parent orientation meeting.

Parent Consultations

The FRC staff should be available for drop-in consultations on any family-related issue. It is important to establish regular hours, so that both parents and teachers can make use of resources. Depending on the culture of the school and referral patterns, this may be a daily activity. Such consultations may be as simple as how to make the homework routine go smoothly, or they may address more serious clinical issues.

Occasionally, students may seek advice from the FRC staff. For instance, a group of girls brought in a friend because they were concerned that she was eating too little. The goal of these consultations is to encourage family-centered solutions. Typically, we recommend that student problem solving be in the hands of the school counselor, because that is the counselor's identified role. If student contact is made, encourage the student to allow contact with parents, and also inform the school counselor to keep up collaborative school relations. Of course, when the student is in imminent danger, contact with the responsible parent is mandatory, and students will need to be apprised of this fact. Point out that it is in the best interests of the student to have the parent involved in solving the problem. It is often helpful to have videotapes and materials of interest to students, to encourage their interest in solving family problems constructively.

Family transitions, divorce, remarriage, change in living situations, and death have all been common concerns of the families we have seen. Divorce and stepparenting are major family stressors with which many families cope effectively. During these transition times, however, consultation and support are often needed. Given that 50%

of the family population experiences divorce, and a large subset of those remarry, it is essential that videotapes, books, and Parent Nights focus on these issues. A modicum of support during stressful times can prevent or reduce harm to the student and family. Videotapes and books on issues of stepparenting and managing the stress of divorce should be available in the FRC library.

Many families seek advice on how to reestablish a good parent–child relationship after a period of time in which either the parent or the child has been out of the home. We are currently working on developing materials dealing with this transition. Many good texts and community resources also exist for the large population of students and families in high-risk urban settings, who deal with loss as a result of violence. Additionally, good community resources usually are available for families who have experienced the death of a family member.

Based on our experience, you can expect that families who receive consultations average about two meetings. We find that diverse families use the FRC resources both voluntarily and when referred. Families come for a variety of family and adolescent problems. In the middle schools, the largest percentage of concerns are about homework, school attendance, and behavior problems. The next most common areas of concern are behavior management problems, communication, and parent–adolescent relationships. Peer conflicts at school and supervision (unsupervised time with peers) are also common themes. Families appear to be comfortable bringing a wide range of issues to the FRC (grief, stepparenting, and drug and alcohol problems). Parental concerns can lead to offering Parent Nights on specific issues or school problem situations.

Parent Nights are received well, lead to good information exchange, and build coalitions and parental networks. We developed Parent Nights on the topics of homework and supervision of peers. When collaboration with school staff is strong, the meetings are well attended. In one middle school, parents agreed to meet regularly on their own to exchange information about peer activities. These parents were proactively identified by school staff, based on their child's participation in a group of peers who spent a lot of unsupervised time together after school. Following from our ecological model, discussions of supervision included developing a list of neighborhood "hot spots." These were areas that parents, police, and school staff identified as places where troubled kids congregate. Parent Nights may also lead to follow-up appointments and the FCU.

Parental Contingencies

If the FRC is established within a well-organized school ecology, it may be possible to provide school-based contingencies for parental collaboration and involvement. School staff often use school suspension, expulsion, after-school detention, pull-out programs, and other ineffective means to reduce student problem behavior. Clearly, expelling young people from the public school setting and sending them to alternative school settings may exacerbate the problem behavior in the long run (see Dishion, McCord, & Poulin, 1999). In some schools, suspensions and expulsions could be withheld, if parents are actively engaged in the FRC services.

To this end, school-based contingencies for parental involvement in the FRC resources are critical. Consistent with a community reinforcement approach, it is often necessary to provide incentives to engage families in need of intervention, due to the chaos and competing demands on their motivation (Azrin, 1970). Figure 9.3 summarizes

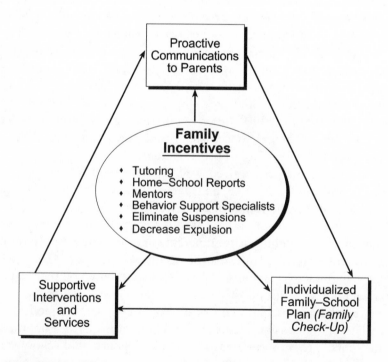

FIGURE 9.3. Engaging parents in a contingent cycle of school and community success.

how consultations with FRC staff, including the FCU and other empirically based intervention services, can be rewarded within a school system.

All schools have "report cards" that contain some information on student behavior, motivation, and citizenship. Contact with the FRC could be initiated by low ratings from teachers on citizenship, discipline referrals, and other concrete behaviors that occur in the school setting. All middle schools, for example, have parent–teacher conferences. In this setting, parents can be informed proactively that students with low citizenship ratings by teachers will meet with both the teacher and FRC staff during parent conference time. The possibility of an individualized student success plan can be discussed with parents, and involves commitments from the student, parent, teacher, and other school staff. The FCU can provide the assessment and collaborative set upon which the plan is based. Examples of plans can be offered on a level system, with Level 1 being a structured weekly report on student attendance (including tardiness), behavior, and homework completion. A Level 2 system might include daily or biweekly feedback to parents on these dimensions, or perhaps, some specialized concerns of either the family or the school.

Given an individualized plan and parental commitment, the potential resources shown in Figure 9.3 can be provided as needed. For instance, the use of mentors is popular with young adolescents. In the Oregon community, the Behavioral Support Specialists were innovated. These mentors are primarily undergraduate students trained to work with high-risk adolescents, using an individualized plan to provide high levels of reinforcement for prosocial behavior. In addition, Behavioral Support Specialists promote skill development to encourage increased success in positive activities. School-based homework support, tutorial support, scholarships to recreational activities, and other community-based incentives enhance high-risk parents' motivation to engage in empirically based support services.

As shown in Figure 9.3, the most innovative schools might consider a contract with parents that guarantees their student will not be suspended or expelled as long as the individualized student plan is being enacted by all. Behavior problems will occur, but they can be anticipated proactively, with school-based consequences provided. A functional assessment of the students' problem behavior in school is the most promising strategy for identifying effective reactions to problem behavior.

Summer Check-Ins

Summertime is probably most convenient for school staff and students, which makes the months of June and September an excellent time to complete the summer check-ins in family homes. Parents often have difficulty with monitoring and time management during the summer months. Checking in with parents and providing information about supervised recreation resources can be extremely valuable to them. We recently developed a summer consultation strategy we refer to as the Next-Year Plan. The service is available for all parents, and they find it extremely useful. Many parents who decline participation in the FCU or other FRC services participate in the Next-Year Plan.

In Appendix B, we provide a checklist for the summer check-ins that focuses on the Next-Year Plan. In collaboration with the FRC staff, parents evaluate the previous year and make commitments for change in the coming school year. Given the high participation by all parents in these brief interventions, it is an excellent opportunity to develop rapport with them and a collaborative set around their goals and concerns for their middle school or high school student.

SUMMARY

In this chapter, we have discussed the goals and activities of the universal level of the FRC. Some problems and possible solutions in establishing the FRC within the typical middle school environment also were discussed.

Although the goals of the FRC are ambitious, we hypothesize that one full-time therapist can have a significant effect on parenting practices in a middle school environment. Presumably, this role could be that of master's-level counselors trained to work collaboratively and effectively with both parents and school staff. We maximize our impact at the universal level by implementing cost-effective universal interventions, such as the SHAPe curriculum, Parent Nights, parent orientation, public-access television, and newsletters to parents. We also suggest training workshops for school staff to improve communication, collaboration, and identification and referral of students and parents.

10

Empirical Support for ATP

In this chapter, we report the main findings on the effectiveness of the components of the multilevel ATP.

The findings described here should not be considered in isolation. There are about 10 active research groups in the world that pioneer and test effective, family-based interventions and prevention strategies. A recent special issue of *Prevention Science* (Spoth, Kavanagh, & Dishion, 2002) highlights several family-centered prevention strategies throughout several regions in the Western Hemisphere (Fisher & Ball, 2002; Kumpfer, Alvarado, Smith, & Bellamy, 2002; Olds, 2002; Sanders, Turner, & Markie–Dadds, 2002; Spoth et al., 2002).

The empirical literature supports family-centered interventions to reduce problem behavior in early childhood (e.g., Webster-Stratton 1990), middle childhood (e.g., Patterson, 1974), and adolescence (Alexander & Parsons, 1973; Henggeler et al., 1998; Liddle, 1999; Szapocznik & Kurtines, 1989). The studies and findings in our intervention research agree well with those of other investigators, providing additional support for the model and intervention strategies described in this volume.

THE ATP FIELD EXPERIMENT

In our original components analysis of ATP (Dishion & Andrews, 1995), we tested a multicomponent intervention that included two cognitive-behavioral curricula—one aimed at self-regulation for young adolescents, and the other at family management for parents. Both interventions are administered in a group setting over 12 weeks and use a semistructured format. We randomly assigned 120 high-risk families to intervention modalities: (1) parent only, (2) teen only, (3) parent and adolescent, and (4) self-directed change.

Figure 10.1 summarizes our hypothesis about how the interventions would result in reduced risk for young adolescents. In short, we expected that improvement in the adolescents' self-regulation, and in the parents' family management, would reduce the level of coercive exchanges within the family, which in turn predict less growth in antisocial behavior and substance use. We also expected the families assigned to both the self-regulation and family management group interventions to show the greatest improvement with respect to re-duced parent–child coercion and later problem behavior. These ex-pectations followed directly from the initial findings and models from the Oregon Youth Study (Dishion et al., 1988).

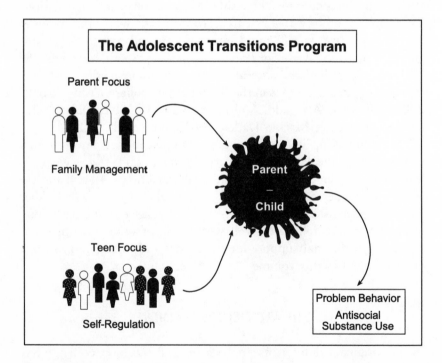

FIGURE 10.1. Hypothesis: How interventions result in reduced risk for young adolescents.

Intervention research is a high-risk enterprise, primarily because the guiding hypotheses are more likely to be unequivocally falsified (Meehl, 1978). Paradoxically, it is rare that an intervention outcome study reports no effects, or worse, negative effects. When unexpected or null effects are found, investigators often attribute the findings to poor measurement (and therefore neglect the measures that render disconfirming data) or poor implementation. These are variations on the theme described by the "file drawer problem": Null or negative findings stay in the file drawer (Dawes, 1994; Landman & Dawes, 1982). Unfortunately, the field grows slowly when negative and null findings are suppressed or omitted from research reports.

This chapter reflects an effort to disclose our full range of findings, as the positive, null, and negative effects have shaped the current version of ATP described in this volume. We organize this discussion into three sections: (1) measurement issues, describing some of the complexities of measuring change among adolescents and their families; (2) bad news, detailing findings that were the opposite of what we expected at the outset; and (3) good news, summarizing positive effects data.

Measurement Issues

Two sets of findings may be useful to consider before reporting the substantive results to the initial multicomponent study. First, we found parents to be highly reactive in their reports of problem behavior. We used the CBCL and PDR as measures of adolescent problem behavior (Chamberlain & Reid, 1987). To recruit our sample of high-risk families, we used community advertisements to elicit parents' telephone calls to the research center. We then screened our sample over the telephone, using the 10 risk factors identified by Bry (1982) to determine which youth would eventually use multiple substances. To ensure that we had an "at-risk" sample, and not a treatment sample, we also stipulated that the young adolescents had *not* been arrested.

There is some evidence that parents adjust their reports of behavior problems at intake in order to ensure a place in the intervention study. We found that all parents reported massive decreases in adolescent problem behavior from baseline and termination on both the CBCL and the PDR measures (Dishion & Andrews, 1995). For example, we excluded a 12-year-old who had been arrested by the police, because we were relatively sure that group interventions would be less effective for the more serious early-onset delinquents (Bank et al., 1991). Moreover, when we actually examined the records of the youth in our study, we found that 28% had records of police contact, despite parental reports of no arrest.

The models on which the interventions were based used a multitrait, multimethod measurement strategy (Campbell & Fiske, 1959; Dwyer, 1983). When using this strategy with passive longitudinal data, we did not worry about the change properties of each of the measures. Eddy, Dishion, and Stoolmiller (1998) reported the unexpected problems we encountered when analyzing change with multitrait, multimethod data. In short, it appears that each person, and each measure, responds uniquely to the demands of an intervention outcome study. Parent, youth, and staff reports of change in monitoring from baseline to termination, for example, were virtually uncorrelated.

In addition to the lack of correlation of change scores, other complexities are encountered with change in problem behavior over time. During adolescence, problem behavior is often thought of as a one-dimensional syndrome. This model fits the data when considering data from one point in time, but fits poorly when considering change data. We factor-analyzed the slopes of individual items on the externalizing scale of the CBCL and found that the change scores produced two factors: behaviors reflecting antisocial behavior, and behaviors reflecting adolescent problem behavior. The former decreased with age, and the latter increased with age (Eddy et al., 1998). The two-factor analytic scales were consistent with Achenbach's (1992) description of the aggressive and delinquency scales, respectively. It turns out that the distinction between these two scales helped us see that our two intervention components were actually affecting adolescents in different ways.

The Bad News

Early in our analyses of the outcome data, we began to see that the young adolescents who were randomly assigned to groups seemed to escalate more on some forms of problem behavior (e.g., self-reported tobacco use and teacher-reported delinquent behavior) than did the control group (Dishion & Andrews, 1995; Dishion, Andrews, et al., 1996). We hoped these effects would be short-lived, but they were not. We found a consistent trend toward increased growth in self-reported tobacco use and teacher-reported delinquent behavior 3 years after the 3-month intervention trial.

Poulin et al. (2001) used latent growth modeling to consider whether this growth in tobacco use and delinquent behavior was statistically associated with the group intervention. As can be seen in Figure 10.2, differences between youth in intervention groups and the control group emerged immediately at termination and were maintained over the course of 3 years.

Negative effects secondary to treatments are often referred to as iatrogenic. Initially, we were concerned that iatrogenic effects were unique to our study, and that a report of negative findings would be irresponsible. However, we discovered other intervention outcome studies that reported similar findings. For example, Lipsey (1992) reported that 29% of all the delinquency intervention studies showed negative effect sizes. What was unclear from the studies, however, was the extent to which the treatments aggregated high-risk adolescents.

A noteworthy exception is the work of Joan McCord in her reports of the Cambridge–Somerville youth study (McCord, 1978, 1981, 1992), probably the most highly controlled field experiment conducted to prevent delinquency among high-risk adolescents. Over 400 youth were matched in pairs on a variety of demographic, behavioral, and physical factors before the intervention began. For each pair, one youth was randomly selected as a control, and the other as an experimental. In the experimental group, the intervention team engaged the youth and family for 4 years in the best possible forms of social work available at that time. The experiment ended when the United States entered World War II.

Thirty years after the intervention, the results were modestly negative. Youth exposed to the massive social work intervention were worse off than those who had been left alone in the control group. These findings became classic in the criminological literature but were virtually ignored in psychology (McCord, 1978).

At the time we were finding the iatrogenic effects for the ATP adolescent groups, we collaborated with McCord to determine if the iatrogenic effects observed in the Cambridge–Somerville youth study were due to aggregating youth. In her reanalysis of these data, she found that youth sent to summer camps on two successive occasions accounted for much of the negative effects observed in this study

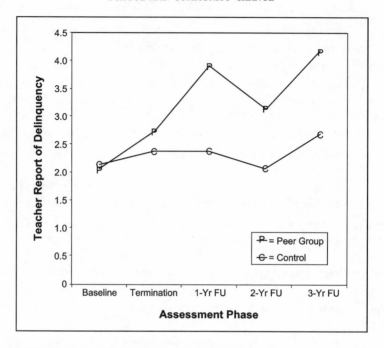

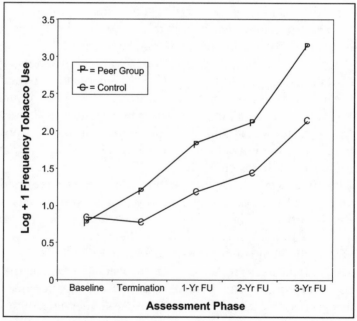

FIGURE 10.2. Simultaneous, two-group analysis of iatrogenic growth in delinquent behavior in school and tobacco use.

(McCord, 1997). These youth had an odds ratio of 10:1 for experiencing negative life outcomes compared to their matched control. These data, as reported in our joint report (Dishion, McCord, & Poulin, 1999), are summarized in Figure 10.3.

The final step in our analysis of iatrogenic effects was to understand which aspects of the groups were associated with the negative effect. In our intervention research, we videotaped every group session for all participating youth. These videotapes assist in providing supervision and conducting post hoc analysis of intervention effects, such as those reported on parenting groups in Chapter 7 (Hogansen & Dishion, 2001). The results are summarized in Figure 10.4.

Basically, we found that a pattern of deviancy training in the groups was associated modestly with negative growth in smoking and problem behavior in school. This was surprising, because we supervised group sessions both to reduce the level of deviant talk in the groups and to promote positive peer support for prosocial behavior and adherence to the cognitive-behavioral curriculum. However, close inspection of the videotapes did reveal surreptitious interactions among the youth during the group sessions, as well as subtle support for deviant talk during unstructured time (before and after the group sessions and during the break).

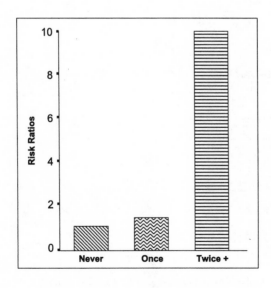

FIGURE 10.3. Bad outcomes associated with attending summer camp.

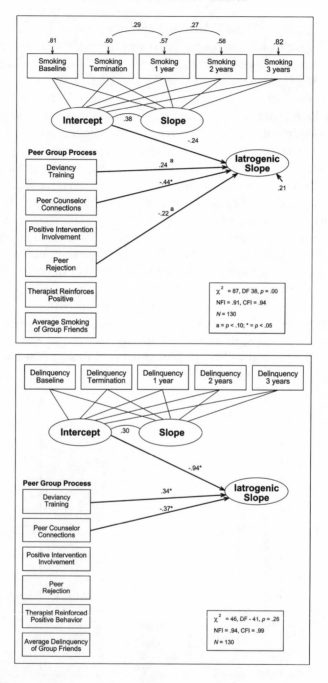

FIGURE 10.4. Predicting iatrogenic growth in self-reported smoking and teacher-reported delinquency from observed peer-group process.

On the plus side, we found that a positive relationship with peer counselors in the group related to less growth in problem behavior. For each of the groups, we selected older high school students to assist in the delivery of the curriculum and to model prosocial skills.

Our conclusion (based on our findings, findings of the Cambridge–Somerville youth study, and other studies reviewed by Dishion, McCord, et al., 1999) is that aggregating youth into groups *potentially* exacerbates their problem behavior. Originally, we hypothesized that it was the aggregation of high-risk youth. Now, however, we suspect that any group treatment in which youth gain attention or develop relationships organized around deviance potentially produces negative effects that are enduring.

Inspection of the videotapes of our groups revealed that even therapeutic moments, in which young adolescents talk about stopping their use of drugs or improving their behavior, contain a significant element of deviancy training (Dishion et al., 1997; Dishion, Andrews, et al., 1996; Dishion, Spracklen, et al., 1996). These discussions capture the attention and interest of all group members, high or low risk. Being the center of attention in a process of showcasing problem behavior seems to be powerfully reinforcing.

Of note, many interventions for adolescents in trouble involve aggregation and low supervision. Observational research in institutional settings suggests that it is virtually impossible for adults to compete with peers in providing reinforcement for prosocial behavior. Buehler and Patterson (1966) found that for every one positive behavior reinforced by an adult, nine deviant behaviors were reinforced by peers in a correctional setting. Clearly, salience of the peer group in adolescence and the dynamics of an institutional setting appear to be the perfect training conditions for creating a serious career criminal or substance abuser.

The Good News

It may well be that the most important results of the first phase of our field experiment were the unanticipated iatrogenic effects. Positive effects—those that we had anticipated and for which we hoped—were also informative. Like many other researchers, we found that interventions focusing on family management were the most cost-effective strategy for reducing escalation in problem behavior among high-risk young adolescents. Along with this finding, we also found that the adolescent intervention was effective for some outcomes.

Our most trusted measure of clinical outcome is direct observations of parent–child interaction. In this study, we asked all adolescents and parents to discuss real-life problems on videotape, according to the procedures adopted by a variety of family researchers (Forgatch, 1989; Robin & Foster, 1989). We then coded the videotapes with the Family Process Code (FPC; Dishion, Gardner, Patterson, Reid, & Thibodeaux, 1983). In the past, as in the present, the focus was the occurrence of coercive interactions. We captured parent–adolescent coercion with a negative engagement score, which reflected the rate per minute of negative exchanges during 25 minutes of videotaped problem solving.

We found that both the self-regulation and the FMC were associated with reductions in parent–child coercion. The average level of negative engagement is summarized in Table 10.1. These data are not only interesting from an intervention outcome perspective but also descriptively. The rate-per-minute scores are readily translated to action. A rate per minute of .5 indicates that for every 2 minutes, a family member engages in one negative behavior. Negative behaviors predominantly include criticism (negative verbal, verbal attack) and, less often, coercive threats or negative physical engagement.

We also found that the teachers reported less antisocial behavior for youth who were randomly assigned to the FMC. As reported in Chapter 6, we found that changes in coercive interactions were associated with reductions in teacher ratings of antisocial behavior, as suggested in Figure 10.1. These results are reported in detail in our first publication of findings (Dishion & Andrews, 1995).

We also examined the impact of the family intervention on subsequent substance use. We found that for the first year following our intervention, the parent-only condition nearly eliminated the onset of smoking, as reported by both the youth and the parent. The effects were similar for the less frequent alcohol and marijuana use but were not statistically reliable (Dishion, Spracklen, et al., 1996). Unfortunately, however, the effects of substance use for the parent intervention faded at 1-year follow-up and thereafter.

The intervention effects for the parent-focused FMC were replicated by Irvine, Biglan, Metzler, Smolkowski, and Ary (1999). These investigators randomly assigned high-risk rural families to a wait-list

TABLE 10.1. Observed Mother and Child Negative Engagement in Family Problem Solving by Intervention Condition and Phase

	Baseline			Termination		
Intervention condition	n	M	(SD)	n	M	(SD)
Mother						
Parent only	24	0.63	(0.63)	23	0.39	(0.44)[a]
Teen only	31	0.67	(0.85)	31	0.52	(0.59)[a]
Parent and teen	31	0.56	(0.81)	29	0.46	(0.47)[a]
Self-directed	27	0.49	(0.51)	25	0.56	(0.84)
Control	39	0.62	(0.54)	35	0.90	(0.89)
Child						
Parent only	26	1.27	(1.33)	24	0.81	(0.88)[a]
Teen only	32	1.09	(1.28)	32	0.80	(0.89)[b]
Parent and teen	31	1.33	(1.58)	31	0.93	(1.09)[a]
Self-directed	27	0.78	(0.82)	25	1.06	(1.32)
Control	39	1.22	(1.14)	35	1.36	(1.53)

Note. Scores refer to the rate per minute of observed behavior.
[a] Statistically reliable positive intervention effect at termination in contrast to controls.
[b] Statistically marginal ($p < .10$) intervention effect in contrast to controls.

control and the FMC. They found that the FMC was associated with improved child-rearing practices (O'Leary, 1995) and reduced problem behavior in the youth. The long-term effects were unexamined because of the wait-list control design.

Conclusions

Our first phase of intervention research provided powerful lessons in the use of intervention research to test developmental models for adolescent problem behavior (Dishion & Patterson, 1999). We learned that the measurement of change is complicated, especially because unique perspectives of reporting agents seem to be differentially reactive to intervention experiment. These issues are, of course, discussed at length in basic texts on psychological experimentation (Campbell & Stanley, 1963; Cook & Campbell, 1979). Future intervention trials should be careful to disentangle measurement effects from reactions to assessment.

We also drew conclusions about the utility of adolescent and parent group intervention strategies for preventing problem behavior, summarized in Figure 10.5.

Basically, these data and a vast literature on child and adolescent problem behavior suggest that interventions aggregating peers are potentially harmful, or at best, ineffective, and those that target parenting practices are beneficial, especially for high-risk families. Given the 1-year duration of intervention effects, we suspect that when working with families of adolescents, booster sessions and continued support may be needed throughout adolescence to guard against the escalating influence of peers from early to middle adolescence (Chassin, Presson, & Sherman, 1990; Dishion, Andrews, et al., 1996).

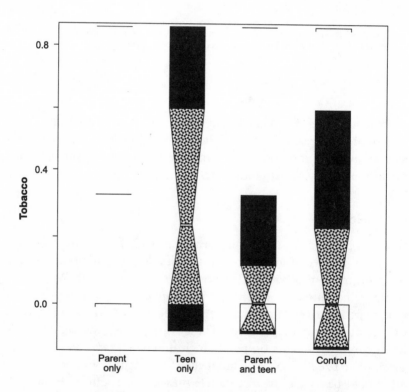

FIGURE 10.5. Monthly tobacco use by intervention condition.

PUBLIC SCHOOL INTEGRATION

Background

Clinical researchers are beginning to document the weakness in testing intervention strategies in university and research institute clinics. Interventions designed within such research contexts produce moderate effect sizes, whereas those implemented in community settings drop to zero (Weiss, Catrone, Harris, & Phung, 1999; Weisz, Weiss, Hahn, Granger, & Morten, 1995).

With this issue in mind, we began a series of studies examining the effectiveness of ATP when implemented within the school context. The pilot experiment involved 60 families randomly assigned to either ATP at school or at our research center. Unfortunately, this study was designed prior to collection of outcome data for our earlier research, in which we ultimately found the iatrogenic effects. Consequently, we included both the parent and adolescent group intervention, in which the inclusion of the adolescent group intervention completely undermined the detection of a parent intervention effect, which speaks to the power of peers in early adolescence.

We did find, however, that the school intervention was modestly more superior than the ATP implemented at the research center (Dishion, Andrews, et al., 1996). It also appears that the iatrogenic effects were fewer when implemented in the school context. This reduction in negative effects may be due either to the inclusion of familiar peers in the adolescent groups or to our efforts to reintegrate the high-risk youth with low-risk youth after the 3-month intervention. These data suggested that our efforts to integrate family-centered interventions within the school context were a step in the right direction.

Project Alliance

In 1994, we explored the possibility of fully integrating ATP within a public school context. The authors worked weekly in an FRC in a public middle school. We attended weekly school staff meetings and served families referred by the counselors and vice principals. Over the next 3 years, we supervised several graduate students in elementary, middle, and high school FRCs. These experiences led to the development of the intervention model described in Chapter 2, and our ideas about working within a school ecology in Chapter 9.

In 1996, the National Institute on Drug Abuse (NIDA) funded the Project Alliance prevention trial to test our ideas. In this study, we randomly assigned two cohorts of sixth-grade youth to a family-enhanced middle school experience (using the multilevel framework). The project was conducted in collaboration with the Portland Public Schools (Oregon). Three middle schools agreed to collaborate in Project Alliance.

The schools graciously assigned homeroom classrooms in agreement with our individual random assignment to intervention or control groups. The first cohort began in 1997 and the second, in 1999. In total, 999 families and their sixth-grade students agreed to participate in our school-based assessment. As of this writing, the second cohort is just completing ninth grade, so our ability to evaluate the long-term impact of the family-based intervention on substance abuse is limited.

Effects on Early Substance Use

We have examined the effects of the ATP multilevel model on adolescent substance use for our first Project Alliance cohort ($n = 672$). The demographics of the sample are summarized in Table 10.2.

Our initial analysis of effectiveness focused on adolescent self-

TABLE 10.2. Gender and Ethnic Composition by Group

	Female				Male			
	ATP		Control		ATP		Control	
Self-identified ethnic group	n	(%)	n	(%)	n	(%)	n	(%)
European American	65	(40.9)	58	(35.8)	71	(41.3)	84	(46.9)
African American	53	(33.3)	53	(32.7)	60	(34.9)	51	(28.5)
American Indian	3	(1.9)	4	(2.5)	5	(2.9)	3	(1.7)
Hispanic American	10	(6.3)	15	(9.3)	13	(7.6)	11	(6.1)
Asian American	12	(7.5)	10	(6.2)	7	(4.1)	8	(4.5)
Pacific Islander	1	(0.6)	2	(1.2)	0	(0.0)	1	(0.6)
European African American	8	(5.0)	17	(10.5)	9	(5.2)	11	(6.1)
Other	7	(4.4)	3	(1.8)	7	(4.1)	10	(5.6)

reports of substance use at grades 6, 7, 8, and 9. We asked the youth to report the number of times they used tobacco, alcohol, marijuana, and other illicit drugs over the previous month. For basis of comparison, we summarized the substance use from sixth grade (first year of middle school) to ninth grade (first year of high school) for both the at-risk and typically developing adolescents. As can been seen in Figure 10.6, self-reports of drug use in middle school are not normally distributed, especially for the typically developing students.

Visual inspection of the data in Figure 10.6 suggests that the intervention effect for the ATP program is strongest for the first year of high school. Logistic regression analyses confirm this impression. When predicting substance use in grade 9, controlling for substance use in grades 6, 7, and 8, the intervention condition produced a reliable reduction for both typically developing and high-risk students. Given that a majority of the FCU and family management interventions were given to high-risk families, these data suggest that the universal component was indeed effective for preventing early-onset substance use by high school for typically developing students. These findings are summarized in detail by Dishion, Kavanagh, et al. (2002).

These analyses suggest that the multilevel, family-centered intervention does provide a preventive effect on self-reported substance use, and that the highest risk youth are the most likely to benefit. Note that the intervention effects did not vary significantly by ethnicity (African American vs. European American) or gender. These data are particularly interesting when considering the amount of contact we had with families during middle school (the data are summarized in Table 10.3).

The average number of professional contacts (including telephone contacts) was 13 for at-risk students and 7 for the typically developing students. In-person time came to 5.6 hours for at-risk and 3.1 hours for the typically developing students. Note that the most contact, by far, was by telephone, with at-risk families receiving a total of slightly less than 2 hours of telephone contact, compared to about 45 minutes for the typically developing families. Compared to other treatment and prevention programs, it appears the ATP model is quite reasonable with respect to the overall amount of professional time and effort.

Over the past decade, we learned a great deal about issues of working with families within a public school environment. There are

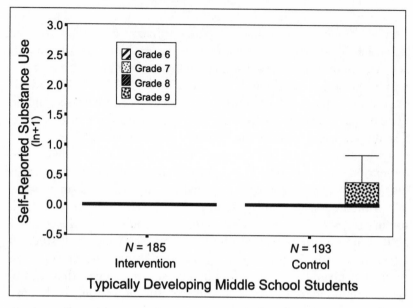

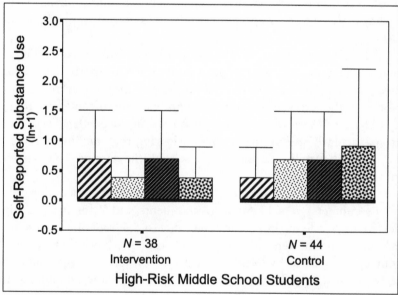

FIGURE 10.6. Self-reported substance use for Project Alliance for typically developing and at-risk students.

TABLE 10.3. Teacher Report of Students' Deviant Peers Regressed on Ethnicity/ Gender, Self-Report of Deviant Peers, Peer Report of Deviant Peers, and GPA

	Unstandardized coefficient		Standardized coefficient		
	β	SE	β	t	p
(Constant)	2.95	0.18	—	16.23	0.00
European American girls	−0.33	0.13	−0.12	−2.52	0.01
European American boys	−0.34	0.12	−0.13	−2.89	0.00
African American girls	−1.34	0.13	−0.05	−1.07	0.29
Self–report of deviant peers	2.01	0.01	0.08	2.25	0.03
Peer report of deviant peers	6.01	0.01	0.32	8.29	0.00
Grade point average (GPA)	−0.48	0.05	−0.36	−9.05	0.00

a number of systemic barriers to implementing empirically based interventions within existing service delivery systems (Hoagwood & Koretz, 1996). First of all, it takes time to establish a new service that gets used by both school staff and parents within a public school system. Second, random assignment at the individual level actually undermines engaging in schoolwide communication practices that are necessary to engage parents to collaborate with school staff. Third, a multiple-gating strategy for identifying high-risk youth may do more harm than good in building a community of family and school, especially for minority families. Finally, students move from school to school: What makes a coherent program in one school actually only meets the needs of the minority of youth in North America who remain in that one middle school. We now discuss each of these issues in detail, as well as potential solutions.

SOME CAVEATS

Time and Reputation

In our early work within public schools, we noticed tremendous variability in usage of the FRC. With a new program, referrals to the FRC are completely dependent on school staff and the ability of school staff to mobilize a family-centered perspective into school behavior management practices. For example, to successfully establish the first FRC in our pilot work, we volunteered for 2 years as parent consultants, attending the weekly behavior management staff meetings. After 2 years, nearly all discipline contacts were referred to the FRC. In another middle school, the FRC received few parent referrals, and FRC personnel had little to do when staffing the room except meet with individual students. In this school, the principal had excellent rapport with parents, and was reluctant to refer parents to FRC resources.

Parents should be familiar with an intervention resource before they agree to participate. For instance, in our first cohort, we were surprised that only 30% of the families who had actually been assessed were interested in receiving feedback on their assessment using the FCU model. However, in Cohort 2, we had 70% of families agree to receive feedback. We presume that two factors may account for this difference: (1) By the beginning of the Cohort 2 process, the parents were more likely familiar with the Project Alliance name and services within the FRC; and (2) in Cohort 2, we began visiting families at the end of the summer to introduce ourselves personally and to inform them of FRC services.

The Science Problem

Another issue is the integration of the needs of science and those of working in service delivery systems. The gold standard of experimental design is to randomly assign individuals to an intervention group and a control group. Especially with a large sample, this random assignment at the individual level ensures that if there are factors competing with our intervention, we can explain the differences found between the intervention and control groups at some later point in time.

In the context of a highly controlled environment, this may be desirable. Random assignment in Project Alliance prevented our FRC staff from a variety of activities that had the potential to increase parent engagement: (1) attending and participating in schoolwide meetings that drew a large number of parents, (2) repeated exposure of the FRC in the school newsletter, and (3) use of television as a medium to connect families within middle schools.

The Next Generation, our current project in Eugene, Oregon, uses a quasi-experimental design, in which we have paired middle schools that feed into the same high school. One school in each pair has the FRC. We are now able to engage in a variety of schoolwide activities to increase parent participation in the FRC activities. We also can link with schoolwide discipline plans to collaborate proactively with parents at an early stage of the escalation process.

Multiple Gating

In the 1980s, we designed a multiple-gating procedure to identify high-risk students cost-effectively. The two-step procedure was designed empirically, considering the predictive validity of each "gate" or screening procedure, following the guidelines for establishing a multistage screening procedure (see Cronbach & Glesar, 1965).

Our screening procedure began with teacher ratings, then parent ratings, and finally, as the third screen, an assessment of family functioning (Loeber & Dishion, 1987; Loeber et al., 1984). More recently, we have discovered that a two-gate procedure is as effective as a three-gate procedure (Dishion & Patterson, 1993).

With Project Alliance, we found other concerns beside predictive validity in our use of teacher ratings as a proactive screening measure. Kavanagh, Burraston, et al. (2000) systematically analyzed the relation between teacher ratings of risk and other indices of problem behavior, including school records, peer nominations, and self-report. Unfortunately, they found a bias in the data: Ethnicity status accounted for unique variance in teacher ratings, after controlling for all other sources of information about the students' problem behavior. Basically, a statistically reliable tendency showed that teachers inadvertently rate African American or nonwhite males at higher risk for problem behavior. Note that approaching parents of these youth to collaborate proactively on reducing risk would clearly be experienced as offensive by those parents. The data are summarized in Table 10.4.

At this stage, we have abandoned teacher ratings as a screening measure, but we have two other recommendations. First, when beginning the implementation of the FRC, a committee of parents and school staff should convene to decide collectively how the FRC will fit within the school system. Every school is unique with respect to grading policies and procedures. Parents may wish to have more specific information on the ABC report cards (e.g., percentage of homework assignments completed, attendance, tardiness) and ratings on specific behaviors (e.g., being on task in class and following school

TABLE 10.4. Level of Engagement by Risk Status

	Family type				
	TD (n = 222)		AR (n = 60)		F
Contact method	Mean	(SD)	Mean	(SD)	(1,280)
Frequency of contact	6.70	(8.40)	13.10	(16.90)	16.48
Total in-person time (hours)	3.12	(5.26)	5.60	(9.09)	6.46
Total telephone time (minutes)	48.30	(60.80)	108.16	(162.17)	19.99

Note. TD, typically developing; AR, at risk.

rules). Like low grades, poor citizenship can be discussed proactively at parent–teacher conferences, and FRC resources can be provided. Teacher biases in rating behaviors can be reduced by our being more behaviorally specific in the definition of "risk" and "problem behavior" and by collaborating with parents at the onset with respect to these definitions.

American Mobility

We presumed at the beginning of our study that a good proportion of our students would stay in the middle schools associated with our FRC. It turns out that more than 50% of the students transferred by eighth grade. As one might expect, the eighth-grade students with the highest level of problem behavior were the most likely to move.

Mobility certainly presents a challenge to the evaluation of a prevention program embedded within a single school. More important, however, is the broader implication for youth in general. If young adolescents are highly mobile, schools have a limited capacity for making a fundamental, long-term impact on students' academic and behavioral adjustment. We are especially concerned that transitions may undermine progress because of the disruptive effect on social networks, social support, and academic progress. In particular, we notice a tendency for the students with marginal behavioral adjustment to be referred to schools that aggregate other high-risk adolescents. This often can be an immediate solution to the overworked school staff but may actually contribute to an escalating pattern of problem behavior for the adolescents. We see the structural issue of mobility as important to address in the future, in an effort to promote academic and social competence, and to prevent problem behavior among young adolescents.

SUMMARY

In this chapter, we reviewed the data leading to the current version of ATP described in this book. In initial studies, we found that aggregating high-risk youth into groups was associated with negative effects on smoking and problem behavior at school: Youth who were put into groups became more problematic. On the positive side, the family-based intervention was the most effective with respect to reducing parent–adolescent coercive interactions, teacher report of antisocial behavior, and young adolescents' initiation into substance use.

More recently, we studied the impact of the ATP model on more than 600 multiethnic youth in a metropolitan area, over the course of their middle school years (grades 6 to 9). Analyses of substance use revealed that at-risk and typically developing youth were less likely to use drugs by the first year of high school, if they were randomly assigned to the services available from the FRC.

11

Science as a Tool for Change

Science is often thought to be an activity of experts. We are in a time when it seems that to do science, we need million-dollar grants, a team of statisticians, and years of graduate training in research.

Our goal in this chapter is to discuss the use of science in everyday professional activity, as a tool for change. Should we use treatment A or B? This is a question anyone could answer with the right data.

The motivation for answering this question is accountability. Researchers not only require service programs to consume the latest research on intervention effectiveness but they also need to show that their own programs work. In fact, it is certain that to use even an empirically validated program in a community, adjustments need to be made. Research evaluating the effectiveness of empirically validated programs in the actual community suggests that effect sizes drop to zero (Kazdin & Weisz, 1998; Weiss et al., 1999). Clearly, the scientific community is in need of feedback. We need to see whether the community of professionals and families who use our findings benefit from them, or not. To conclude this volume, this chapter provides a brief overview of diverse strategies for evaluating the effectiveness of the kinds of services described in this volume.

PRAGMATICS OF EVALUATING INTERVENTIONS

In considering the ecological cube presented in Chapter 2, three levels of services may require evaluation: (1) clinical interventions with individual adolescents and families, (2) interventions in schools, and (3) community-level interventions. Each is discussed in turn.

INTERVENTIONS WITH FAMILIES

Two basic strategies are used for evaluating the impact of an intervention with a family. The first is periodic data collection to enable the graphing of problem behavior during the course of treatment. The second is a pre- and post-design, more useful for testing the effectiveness of a treatment for an individual family or of an intervention strategy for the purposes of accountability or program evaluation.

For the first strategy, measures are needed that capture key family dynamics and problem behavior under short time frames, so that increases and decreases can be assessed. Standardized rating forms often are not useful, because they involve time frames from 2 to 6 months. We prefer time frames from 1 day to 1 week (Eddy et al., 1998).

We propose the Child Daily Report (CDR) and Parent Daily Report (PDR) as measures to use in the course of evaluating the impact of an intervention program for a family. The measures are described in Chapter 3, along with norms for normative and high-risk families with young adolescents. The telephone reports are cost-effective assessment strategies that are relatively inexpensive to collect. Chamberlain and Reid (1987) report that the PDR, in particular, is a useful measure of change, especially when the clinical concerns of the parents are included in the list of problem behavior and tracked for change.

As discussed in Chapter 10, the problem with exclusive reliance on the PDR is that, under some conditions, parents may overreport improvement (Dishion & Andrews, 1995). However, this problem may be minimal when parents are not required to qualify for a treatment service by reporting initial high levels of problem behavior. A weekly or biweekly assessment of the PDR of "targeted" behavior problems can be an especially useful strategy in service settings that are not externally funded for evaluation.

By way of example, we examined the problem behavior of 4 American Indian adolescents living in reservation communities (see Figure 11.1). The 4 youth and their families were referred to an Indian health services clinic serving the reservation communities. In working with each family, we conducted an Indian Family Wellness Intervention (Dionne, 1997), an adaptation of the Family Check-Up

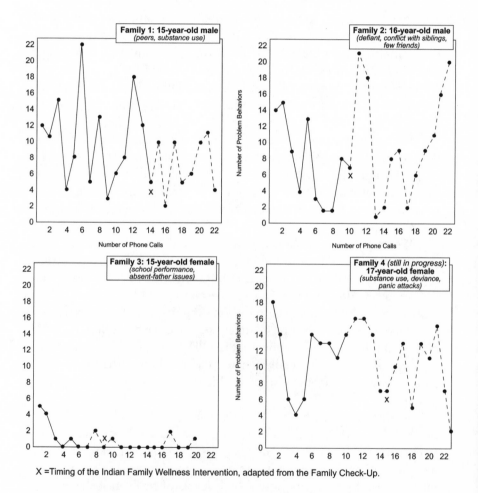

X =Timing of the Indian Family Wellness Intervention, adapted from the Family Check-Up.

FIGURE 11.1. Four families involved in family intervention.

(FCU), to address historical trauma of American Indian families (Duran & Duran, 1995). The three-session intervention had a noticeable impact on reducing problem behavior in 2 of the adolescent youth: One appeared to engage in few problem behaviors in the home context, whereas the other's problem behavior seemed to escalate somewhat following the brief intervention.

The PDR data certainly would suggest that the family whose problems escalated could benefit from a review and potentially more intensive family support. In this particular family, the father had a severe alcohol problem but refused involvement in the family intervention.

The second research strategy is to conduct a pre- and post-measure of outcome for each family. For this, many of the available clinical outcome measures can be useful as long as the time frame is adjusted to match the length of treatment. We propose the use of an observation task for evaluating the effectiveness of a family-centered intervention to change the family interaction patterns. In our briefest assessment, we use the observed family problem-solving task, also described in Chapter 3. With respect to program evaluation, changes in family interaction patterns have been linked to changes in more global measures of antisocial behavior (Dishion et al., 1992).

Measuring coercion in family interactions is not as difficult as it seems. We developed a brief, inexpensive, time-sampling approach to measuring family coercion and positive parenting practices that we refer to as the Relationship Process Code (RPC; Dishion, Rivera, Jones, Verberkmoes, & Patras, 2002). Training in the use of the RPC is relatively easy, and the code can be used in most clinical settings.

When examining change, it is possible to quantify the level of change for each case, addressing whether a family has made statistically reliable change, clinically significant change, or both (Jacobsen & Truax, 1991). To examine whether the changes observed in an individual family are statistically reliable, we compare the pre- and postmeasures, and divide by the standard error of measurement. A t score of 2.00 (– or +) reflects statistically reliable change. Clinically significant change suggests that a client went from the distress range to the normative range of functioning. To calculate clinically significant change, estimate the means and standard deviations for families considered "distressed" (or high-risk) and those considered "normative" (see Jacobsen & Truax, 1991, for details). The data in Chapter 3 can be used to calculate clinically significant change for individual families on measures we developed for ATP.

SCHOOL INTERVENTIONS

In beginning our research on the ATP, we were convinced that in order to evaluate an intervention, relationship interactions must be directly observed. This assumption makes it difficult to evaluate interventions designed to impact larger systems and populations. We now believe that there are less expensive and more valid strategies for evaluating the impact of an intervention program. For example, drug-use prevention researchers rely on youth self-report surveys as an indicator of a positive program impact. Random assignment to drug prevention programs reliably produced reductions in tobacco, alcohol, and marijuana use (e.g., Botvin et al., 1990). As discussed in Chapter 10, we found that youth report of substance use showed positive effects for our family-centered intervention (Dishion et al., 2003). Metzler, Biglan, Rusby, and Sprague (2001) found student survey reports of positive teacher–student interactions and perceptions of safety to be sensitive to a schoolwide evaluation of the Effective Behavior Support (EBS) program.

Given that students can be inexpensively assessed in schools, the use of school surveys are ideal. One problem that needs to be addressed, however, is the extent to which student surveys are vulnerable to the Hawthorne effect; that is, student-reported intervention and prevention effects may reflect the demand characteristics of the evaluation. Campbell and Stanley (1963) originally described this as an assessment-by-intervention interaction and a serious threat to the internal validity of the evaluation study.

The other approach that has tremendous ecological validity is to use data collected by the school (e.g., attendance, discipline contacts, referrals, and grades). These data are unobtrusive and inexpensive to collect. Sugai and colleagues (1999) have used this strategy in the development of the EBS program. Metzler et al. (2001) also used this approach to compare EBS results within the experimental school. The drawback to school-record indices of intervention effects is that schools often do not keep careful records. As discussed in Chapter 9, establishing a standard system for collecting attendance and behavioral referral data is an excellent first step in the change process.

COMMUNITY INTERVENTIONS

Biglan and colleagues have encouraged behavioral scientists to think more broadly about the relevance of their work to community change (Biglan, 1995; Biglan, Glasgow, & Singer, 1990). As in all evaluation research, the validity of the science depends on measurement and the ability of the research design to reduce interpretive noise (i.e., alternative explanations).

Measurement is a particularly difficult problem when examining community change. Biglan (1995) proposes that policy affects the systematic collection of prevalence and incidence data on adolescent problem behavior as a matter of course. The Monitor the Future studies funded by the NIDA are an indispensable tool for examining the impact of policy on drug use among U.S. high school students (e.g., O'Malley, Bachman, & Johnston, 1988). Although these are useful data, such surveys that are community-specific would be even more useful. Yearly (or even monthly) reports of adolescent problem behavior in local newspapers could incite community change and the use of sound prevention strategies.

Design issues are complicated when it comes to evaluating communitywide interventions. The quasi-experimental design has certainly been used and provides compelling evidence for communitywide change in response to prevention programs (e.g., Johnson et al., 1990; Pentz et al., 1989). It is no mystery that such studies are expensive and often out of reach for most communities, states, or even countries. More recently, Biglan and Taylor (2000) described the use of a multiple baseline design to evaluate community change. This design integrates the strengths of measurement available in survey research with the repeated-measure designs described in the PDR, with the power of looking at larger social units such as communities. Figure 11.2 provides an overview of how this might work when comparing an intervention impact of four communities within a given state, guiding change in mental health services over the course of 8 years.

Given that resources require some pacing with the implementation of social change, the multiple baseline approach seems particu-

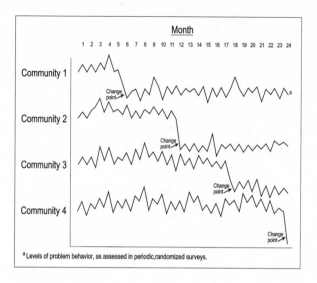

FIGURE 11.2. Evaluating change at the community level.

larly fitting to the evaluation of social policy. For instance, in a state that wants to change its policies toward a family-centered strategy, leaders could randomly assign four communities to participate in the implementation of the policy. Community 1, the first to receive a comprehensive version of ATP, would provide funding and infrastructure for all middle and high schools to develop a Family Resource Center (FRC). Training the therapists to staff the FRCs, and getting the interventions under way, takes at least 2 years per school, so effects would not be observed for 2 or 3 years.

The CDR and PDR could be administered on a monthly basis to a randomly selected sample of students and families from all four communities. Prevalence rates of violence, substance use, and even depression could be estimated. As effects are observed in Community 1, the intervention would move its resources to Community 2 and repeat the process. By the time effects are observed in Community 2, it might be unnecessary to test the effects again, and perhaps the model could be implemented in both Communities 3 and 4. Systematic community change and policy implementation is also science that is both mutually informative and a guide to action that benefits the community, children, and families, and ultimately the leadership that will be held accountable for its efforts, or the lack thereof.

Fisher and Ball (2002) described this approach for use within three Native American communities. Their report is useful because it identifies a process of tribal ownership and participation in both the research process and the intervention design. Using sound principles of community change (Kelly, 1988) and sensitivity in order not to perpetuate historical trauma suffered in those communities (Duran & Duran, 1995), they found high levels of engagement and participation by both families in the community and the tribal leadership. The advantage of the multiple baseline design is that it allows for the organic nature of community change to unfold as it will and, at the same time, provides a useful and ethical framework for evaluating the impact of change efforts. Note that iatrogenic effects, if observed, would justify changing the intervention and preventing the dissemination of strategies that inadvertently do harm.

CONCLUSIONS

Our goal in this book is to provide the culmination of over 15 years of research in applying science to the design of effective and humane interventions for adolescents who are in trouble. Personal and professional experience suggest that teenage problem behavior is more than a short-lived irritant to adults—it can disrupt the course of young people's lives. It seemed an appealing notion that science could help prevent these negative outcomes for those adolescents most at risk (Patterson et al., 1992).

Perhaps the answer is common sense: Adults are needed to guide a young person through the vicissitudes of adolescence and peer networks. One might argue that because the answer *is* common sense, the science was not needed in the first place.

At this juncture, it may be appropriate to underscore how science can continue to contribute to the effort to promote positive adjustment and reduce harm to young people. We have seen several waves of "causal" explanations for teenage problem behavior, ranging from purely biological (e.g., difficult temperament) to environmental (e.g., poor parenting) factors. As always, the truth is less than satisfying: Some children may be more temperamentally susceptible to difficult parenting and peer environments.

Although this proposition may be acceptable, or even predicted by the casual human observer, there are some important details missing that science can provide. First, the interaction processes within the adolescents' troubled lives can only be studied with the use of careful observation procedures with well-developed measurement strategies. Through an accumulation of knowledge resulting from a series of studies that clarify the measurement and developmental dynamics, we arrive at a point of being able to test and rigorously evaluate intervention services within an experimental field trial (Dishion & Patterson, 1999).

We have learned the folly of thinking that a model for the development of adolescent problem behavior guarantees success when applied to the design of an intervention service. If service systems do not attend to the human dynamics underlying social development, they may fail to change behavior, or worse, may cause harm, such as in the finding that aggregating high-risk youth into interventions *increased* the very behavior we wished to decrease. This was *not* common sense, apparently, because aggregating high-risk youth seems to be the favored response of virtually all service settings as of this writing (i.e., school, mental health, and juvenile justice systems).

We must take an honest look at our professional services with respect to the young people and families we serve. As a counterbalance to judgment biases, we need science to check those self-serving perceptions of the utility of our professional and services (Dawes, 1994). To this extent, our work led us into a boundary area with unclear definitions. One area of the science for which we were trained tells us about the "developmental trajectories" of the individual. The other area, the science of "human systems," considers the dynamics of organizations with respect to actions and reactions to mental health services. To guarantee continued progress in preventing and reducing adolescent problem behavior and improving mental health, the science of systems needs to be applied to that of the individual.

Glossary

AIM	Assessment, intervention, and motivation
ASUB	Aggregated substance use
ATP	Adolescent Transitions Program
CBCL	Child Behavior Checklist
CDR	Child Daily Report
COIMP	Coder Impressions
CPI	Coercive Process Index
DSM	*Diagnostic and Statistical Manual of Mental Disorders*
EBS	Effective Behavior Support
FAsTask	Family Assessment Task
FCU	Family Check-Up
FIQ-A	Family Intake Questionnaire—Adolescent Version
FMC	Family Management Curriculum
FMEVE	Family Events Checklist
FMG	Family Management Group
FPC	Family Process Code
FRAMES	Feedback, responsibility, advice, menu, empathy, self-efficacy

FRC	Family Resource Center
HSRULFU	House Rules Follow-Up
KIDSC	Teen Self-Check
M	Means
NIDA	National Institute on Drug Abuse
PARSC	Parent Self-Check
PDR	Parent Daily Report
PPI	Positive Process Index
RPC	Relationship Process Code
RPM	Realistic, under the parents' control, measurable
SANE	See Figure 6.2
SD	Standard deviation
SEK	Standard error of kurtosis
SHAPe	Success, Health, and Peace
SUBST	Parent Substance Use
TDR	Teacher Daily Report
TPRSK	Teacher Perception of Risk

For information about how to obtain a copy of any of these measures or related publications, please go to the Child and Family Center website, *http://cfc.uoregon.edu.*

Guidelines for Writing the Family Check-Up Report

The purpose of the Family Check-Up report is to provide information that supports family change and places parents in the central role of change agent and decision maker. This necessitates that the assessment data be clearly reported, that inferences and recommendations be based on knowledge of best practices, and that suggested interventions be realistic and appropriate to the community.

Families are seeking help voluntarily. It is important for reports to be written in a way that parents can read them and not be insulted or embarrassed. This is not to say that we write for the parents as consumers. However, reports also should be written for other professionals who make use of your professional work and considered judgment.

A list of sections that must be included follows. It is helpful (to you!) that the report be additive. The Family Context and Presenting Problem sections can be written after the intake interview. The Family Assessment and Recommendations sections can be done following the assessment and feedback sessions. Finally, the Feedback Session should represent the information conveyed and the shared understanding between the therapist and parent on future intervention activity.

FAMILY CONTEXT

This section provides an overview of the family, which is separate from the presenting problem. Here are some ideas:

1. *Cultural context* is any information that would help you understand the cultural context of the family. Identify salient features of the family's culture. Describe the ethnic context as specifically as possible, using terms such as combined European American, Hispanic, African American, recently immigrated Russian family, and so forth. Geographical and previous political contexts of family life are often as important to understanding as the family's educational and occupational history.

2. *Family constitution and history* describes the historical structure of the family and can include number of parents or caretakers, siblings and ages, marital transitions, target child's placement in the family, child developmental and problem behavior, school and legal history, and parents' legal, substance use, health, and work histories.

3. *Current family functioning* should include information on present school, legal issues, substance use, health, and employment.

PRESENTING PROBLEM

This section focuses on the primary concerns of the caregiver and adolescent, specific to the family's referral. Begin with a description of the referral problem, incorporating the parents' global report, as well as a behaviorally specific description. For example,

> "Mr. Smith expressed concern over John's behavior for the last 2 months and wonders if it is typical teenage behavior. When queried specifically, he reported concern about John lying, talking back, and frequent problems with both school work and school behavior."

The remainder of this section provides information relevant to the presenting problem. Consider historical information (i.e., developmental history) about the child, the family, or both, that pertains to the presenting problem. Think of this section as a reconnaissance flight over the clinical terrain, which is relevant to the presenting problem. Provide the reader with a sense of the larger issues surrounding barriers and resources to change.

Although an intake report stops with the presenting problem and contextual description, it should be written to assist any professional in targeting the next step that supports the family's efforts to address the presenting problem.

FAMILY ASSESSMENT

Remember that the average professional consumer of your report will not be accustomed to a thorough family assessment, so an overview is helpful.

> "Mr. and Mrs. Smith agreed to participate in a family assessment, which consists of a battery of questionnaires for the parent, teachers at school, and John, and a structured family interaction task. The 45-minute family interaction task was conducted in the home and included a series of tasks that were videotaped and studied."

Measures

The measures used for the family assessment are as follows:

- Teacher Ratings of Peers and Social Skills (TPRSK)
- Parent Ratings of Peers and Social Skills (PPRSK)
- Child Ratings of Peers and Social Skills (CPRSK)
- Videotaped Family Interaction Task (FIT)
- School records of grades and discipline contacts
- Child Behavior Checklist (CBCL); parent, youth, and teacher versions
- Live observation at school
- Family Events Checklist (FMEVE, stress)
- Dyadic Adjustment Scale (DAS, marital)

Many psychological reports are based solely on unstructured interviews, or on tests and assessment procedures that are not validated empirically. It is important for the reader to understand that a family assessment represents considerable, collective work and reflects best practices in mental health service delivery. Make it clear that the statements in your report are based on a personal experience with the family, in conjunction with sound assessment practices.

FEEDBACK SESSION

The outside reader must understand that the parents scheduled another appointment to receive feedback on their assessment. This fact speaks to the parents' commitment to the change process. If problems occurred with cancellations or completing the assessment, these should be discussed as relevant factors to consider in the change process.

In order to reduce the burden of reporting all your assessment findings, this section helps you learn how to summarize your feedback to the family. Parents should not encounter any surprises if they happen to read this section. Cover your feedback on both the strengths and weaknesses. Start with something like the following:

> "Betty and Pete Smith attended the 90-minute feedback session. In this meeting, the major findings of the assessment were discussed, as well as implications for addressing the presenting problem. . . ."

Now, go through the various assessed domains in about three paragraphs. Include the child's behavior at home and school, family management, interaction processes and context, and peer relations.

> "John's behavior at home and school was assessed using the Child Behavior Checklist. At home, the father reported aggressive and delinquent behavior in the clinical range. Betty Smith reported some concerns in these areas, but at a level within normal limits. John self-reported delinquent behavior in the clinical range as well. His homeroom teacher did not report significant behavior problems."

In the written report, it is probably easier to begin with a summary of the strengths and to end with areas of concern. Begin with something like the following:

> "Despite these strengths, the family assessment revealed concerns. . . ."

RECOMMENDATIONS

End the report with a two- to three-sentence summary of your case conceptualization, then add intervention recommendations. In this section, it serves the family to include your professional judgment about the dynamics needed for change and the kinds of supports that might be realistically required.

> "This is a two-parent, six-child family in which the parents have reconciled after a year of being divorced. The parents are motivated and expressed concern about the well-being and behavior of all their children, especially the two sons in middle school. School and parent assessments confirmed their concern, showing clinically significant behavior and academic problems.

"Various courses of action were discussed with Mr. and Mrs. Smith. Because of the multiple family stresses, their current marital transition, and the needs of all six children, it was agreed that a more comprehensive family service was needed. This should include case management services for employment assistance for Mrs. Smith and early intervention and day care for the younger children. . . . "

The report can go on here, depending on the needs of the case. Know that if this is a well-written, professional report, the recommendations could have a significant impact. Schools and some community mental health agencies often take these reports seriously. When you have a sense of your audience and how the recommendations might be received, include a more detailed analysis. For example,

"The Smiths noted that previous attempts to improve John's school behavior have been unsuccessful. It is critical that a change plan be developed in conjunction with the special education services at Hope Middle School, providing Betty Smith with daily information on John's homework, behavior in class, and attendance. A suggestion was made that the parents offer incentives for successful days and that limit-setting for school problems be restricted to the school setting. . . . "

In this hypothetical situation, the family counselor thought the special education staff in this school was in the best position to coordinate the services John needed, which basically came down to daily monitoring and incentives. In another school, the school psychologist, counselor, or vice principal might be identified, based on their role in the school and competence with behavioral plans. An informal discussion with those who might conduct the recommended services can always be helpful in determining whether your suggestions are realistic and acceptable.

Finally, it goes without saying that your report must be put together carefully. Like any well-written document, plan on revising at least once. Check your spelling and grammar. Avoid vague statements or therapy jargon ("The client has unresolved issues" or "unexpressed anger"). A report that contains jargon is poorly written and unprofessional, and will probably be ignored. Professionals who work with children and families all day, every day are less than tolerant of such reports. The goal of the Family Check-Up report, then, is to create a document that maximizes the potential for family change and the collaboration between caregivers, and school personnel, and other professionals.

Next-Year Plan and Summer Check-In

Review of _____ Grade

	Good	Satisfactory	Needs Improvement
✎ Grades	_____	_____	_____
✎ Attendance	_____	_____	_____
✎ Peers	_____	_____	_____
✎ Behavior	_____	_____	_____
✎ Smoking & Other Drugs	_____	_____	_____

Goals/Expectations for _____ Grade
(Be specific!)

◎ Grades _____

_____

◎ Attendance _____

_____

◎ Peers _____

_____

◎ Behavior _____

_____

◎ Drugs _____

_____

Classroom Information

◇?◇ What is the atmosphere/seating arrangement where my child is seated?

◇?◇ What is the method for giving assignments?

◇?◇ What is the procedure for getting assignments that my child failed to write down?

◇?◇ How and when are assignments turned in?

◇?◇ Can assignments be turned in late? How are these graded?

◇?◇ Is the teacher available for help before or after school?

◇?◇ How does the teacher communicate student progress to the parent?

◇?◇ When is a good time for parents to visit or call the teacher?

◇?◇ What are expectations for classroom behavior?

In-Home Support for School Success

☞ Eat meals together?

☞ Child gets at least 8 hours of sleep each night?

☞ Check in each day about school and friends?

☞ Promote the importance of school?
How? _____

☞ Promote the importance of respect toward teachers and fellow
    students?
How? _____

☞ Promote positive child activities/interests?
What? _____

☞ Promote positive ways to handle stress?
How? _____

Grades and Academic Skills Checklist

Instructions: For each skill below, enter a "+" if this is a current strength, "O" if it is okay, and "–" if it is a skill or behavior that needs attention.

Child:

_____ Brings assignments home

_____ Turns assignments in

_____ Organizes time for long-term project

_____ Has all necessary school materials and brings them to school

_____ Studies for tests

_____ Takes tests well

_____ Has good motivation

_____ Comes to class prepared to work

Parent:

_____ Has met all teachers and discussed expectations

_____ Has a daily time for study

_____ Has a quiet place for study

_____ Is present during homework

_____ Stays current on information about school

Totals: +   O   –

      _____   _____   _____

Attendance Checklist

Instructions: For each skill below, enter a "+" if this is a current strength, "O" if it is okay, and "–" if it is a skill or behavior that needs attention.

Child:

_____ Regularly wants to go to school

_____ Gets up easily in the morning

_____ Goes to bed by _____ P.M. and is up by _____.

_____ Doesn't skip classes

_____ Doesn't leave school during classes

_____ Doesn't spend time with other children who skip school

Parent:

_____ Goes to bed after child

_____ Makes sure child is in bed by set time

_____ Makes sure child is up in time for school

Totals: +   O   –

_____   _____   _____

Behavior Checklist

Instructions: For each skill below, enter a "+" if this is a current strength, "O" if it is okay, and "–" if it is a skill or behavior that needs attention.

Child:

_____ Doesn't get into fights

_____ Doesn't get into conflicts with other students

_____ Follows school rules

_____ Shows respect for teachers/other adults at school

_____ Shows respect for other students

_____ Doesn't wander out of class

_____ Follows guidelines for talking in class

_____ Sits still in class

_____ Easily gets into conflicts with adults

Parent:

_____ Talks to school about any problem behavior

_____ Discusses any school problems with child

_____ Offers strategies for handling future problems

Totals: +   O   –

_____   _____   _____

Peers Checklist

Instructions: For each skill below, enter a "+" if this is a current strength, "O" if it is okay, and "–" if it is a skill or behavior that needs attention.

Child:

_____ Doesn't spend class time talking with friends

_____ Doesn't spend time with friends I don't know

_____ Has supportive friends at school

_____ Spends time with children who value school

_____ Doesn't spend time with children who get into trouble

_____ Doesn't spend time at friends' homes unsupervised

_____ Doesn't try to look like a gang member

Parent:

_____ Has met all of child's friends

_____ Talks regularly about activities and conflict with peers

_____ Don't know

Totals: +   O   –

        _____   _____   _____

Drugs Checklist

Instructions: For each skill below, enter a "+" if this is a current strength, "O" if it is okay, and "−" if it is a skill or behavior that needs attention.

Child:

_____ Doesn't use any form of tobacco (smoke, chew, use snuff)

_____ Doesn't use alcohol

_____ Doesn't use other drugs

_____ Doesn't spend time with peers who smoke, drink, or use other drugs

_____ Has a plan for refusing drugs if offered by peers

Parent:

_____ Doesn't smoke

_____ Doesn't use alcohol

_____ Doesn't use other drugs

_____ Has clear rules/expectations about drug use

_____ Talks to parents who are hosting a social event

_____ Gives strategies for handling difficult situations

Totals: +   O   −

_____   _____   _____

_____-Grade Plan

The area we want to improve or maintain is _____.

A. Child:
Pick one or two things you can do each day to keep on track:

1. _____

2. _____

B. Parent:
Identify one or two specific things that you will do. If there are not areas of concern at the present time, you should still identify one or two preventive practices that you can do each day to keep your child on track.

At a minimum, strive for 15 minutes a day that is parent–child time.

1. _____

2. _____

C. Family Resource Specialist:
I will:

1. _____

2. _____

_____	_____	_____
Child	Parent	Family Resource Specialist
_____	_____	_____
Date	Date	Date

References

Achenbach, T. M. (1992). New developments in multiaxial empirically based assessment of child and adolescent psychopathology. In J. C. Rosen & P. McReynolds (Eds.), *Recent advances in psychological assessment* (Vol. 8., pp. 75–102). New York: Plenum Press.

Alexander, J. F., & Parsons, B. V. (1973). Short-term behavioral intervention with delinquent families: Impact on family process and recidivism. *Journal of Abnormal Child Psychology, 81,* 219–225.

Andrews, D. W., Soberman, L. H., & Dishion, T. J. (1995). The Adolescent Transitions Program: A school-based program for high-risk teens and their parents. *Education and Treatment of Children, 18,* 478–484.

Arnold, J., Levine, A., & Patterson, G. R. (1975). Changes in sibling behavior following family intervention. *Journal of Consulting and Clinical Psychology, 43,* 683–688.

Azrin, N. H. (1970). Punishment of elicited aggression. *Journal of Experimental Analysis of Behavior, 14,* 7–10.

Bandura, A. (1997). *Self-efficacy. The exercise of control.* New York: Freeman.

Bank, L., Marlowe, J. H., Reid, J. B., Patterson, G. R., & Weinrott, M. R. (1991). A comparative evaluation of parent training for families of chronic delinquents. *Journal of Abnormal Child Psychology, 19,* 15–33.

Barkley, R. A., Edwards, G., Laneri, M., Fletcher, K., & Metevia, L. (2001). The efficacy of problem-solving communication training alone, behavior management training alone, and the combination for parent–adolescent conflict in teenagers with ADHD and ODD. *Journal of Consulting and Clinical Psychology, 69,* 926–941.

Barriga, A. Q. (1997). Preliminary evaluation of a social-cognitive model of adolescent problem behaviors. *Dissertation Abstracts International: Section B: The Sciences and Engineering, 57,* 4739.

Baumrind, D. (1985). Familial antecedents of adolescent drug use: A developmental perspective. In C. L. Jones & R. J. Battjes (Eds.), *Etiology of drug abuse: Implication for prevention* (Research Monograph No. 56, pp. 13–44). Washington, DC: U.S. Government Printing Office.

Bierman, K. L. (1990). Improving the peer relations of rejected children. In B. B. Lahey & A. E. Kazdin (Eds.), *Advances in clinical child psychology* (pp. 131–149). New York: Plenum Press.

Biglan, A. (1992). Family practices and the larger social context. *New Zealand Journal of Psychology, 21,* 37–43.

Biglan, A. (1995). *Changing cultural practices: A contextualist framework for intervention research.* Reno, NV: Context Press.

Biglan, A., Glasgow, R. E., & Singer, G. (1990). The need for a science of larger social units: A contextual approach. *Behavior Therapy, 21,* 195–215.

Biglan, A., Lewin, L., & Hops, H. (1990). A contextual approach to the problem of aversive practices in families. In G. R. Patterson (Ed.), *Depression and aggression: Two facets of family interactions* (pp. 103–129). New York: Erlbaum.

Biglan, A., & Taylor, T. K. (2000). Increasing the use of science to improve child-rearing. *Journal of Primary Prevention, 21,* 207–226.

Bolstad, O. D., & Johnson, S. M. (1972). Self-regulation in the modification of disruptive classroom behavior. *Journal of Applied Behavior Analysis, 5*(4), 443–454.

Botvin, G. J., Baker, E., Dusenbury, L., Tortu, S., & Botvin, E. M. (1990). Preventing adolescent drug abuse through a multimodal cognitive-behavioral approach: Results of a 3–year study. *Journal of Consulting and Clinical Psychology, 58,* 437–446.

Botvin, G. J., Griffin, K. W., Diaz, T., Scheier, L. M., Williams, C., & Epstein, J. A. (2000). Preventing illicit drug use in adolescents: Long-term follow-up data from a randomized control trial of a school population. *Addictive Behavior, 25,* 769–774.

Brown, J. M., & Miller, W. R. (1993). Impact of motivational interviewing on participation and outcome in residential alcoholism treatment. *Addictive Behaviors, 7,* 211–218.

Bry, B. H. (1982). Reducing the incidence of adolescent problems through preventive intervention: One- and five-year follow-up. *American Journal of Community Psychology, 10*(3), 265–276.

Bry, B., & Canby, C. (1986). Decreasing adolescent drug use and school failure: Long-term effects of targeted family problem-solving training. *Child and Family Behavior Therapy, 8,* 43–59.

Bry, B. H., McKeon, P., & Pardina, R. J. (1982). Extent of drug use as a function of number of risk factors. *Journal of Abnormal Psychology, 91,* 273–279.

Buchanan, C. M., Maccoby, E. E., & Dornbusch, S. M. (1991). Caught between parents: Adolescents' experience in divorced homes. *Child Development, 62,* 1008–1029.

Budney, A. J., Higgins, S. T., Delaney, D. D., Kent, L., & Bickel, W. K. (1991). Contingent reinforcement of abstinence with individuals abusing cocaine and marijuana. *Journal of Applied Behavior Analysis, 24,* 657–665.

Buehler, R. E., & Patterson, G. R. (1966). The reinforcement of behavior in institutional settings. *Behaviour Research and Therapy, 4,* 157–167.

Bullock, B. M., & Dishion, T. J. (2002). Sibling collusion and problem behavior in early adolescence: Toward a process model for family mutuality. *Journal of Abnormal Child Psychology, 30,* 143–153.

Bullock, B. M., & Dishion, T. J. (2003). Conduct disorder. In J. J. Ponzetti (Ed.), *The international encyclopedia of marriage and family relationships* (2nd ed., Vol. 1, pp. 349–354). New York: MacMillian Reference USA.

Cairns, R. B., & Cairns, B. D. (1984). Predicting aggressive patterns in girls and boys: A developmental study. *Aggressive Behavior, 10,* 227–242.

Cairns, R. B., Cairns, B. D., Neckerman, H. J., Ferguson, L. L., & Gariepy, J. L. (1989). Growth and aggression: 1. Childhood to early adolescence. *Developmental Psychology, 25,* 1–30.

Cairns, R. B., Perrin, J. E., & Cairns, B. D. (1985). Social structure and social cognition in early adolescence: Affiliative patterns. *Journal of Early Adolescence, 5,* 339–355.

Campbell, S. B. (1994). Hard-to-manage preschool boys: Externalizing behavior, social competence, and family context at 2–year follow-up. *Journal of Abnormal Child Psychology, 22,* 147–166.

Campbell, D. T., & Fiske, D. W. (1959). Conversant and discriminant validation of the multitrait and multimethod matrix. *Psychological Bulletin, 56,* 81–105.

Campbell, D. T., & Stanley, J. C. (1963). Experimental and quasi-experimental designs for research on teaching. In N. L. Gage (Ed.), *Handbook of research teaching* (pp. 171–246). Chicago: Rand McNally.

Capaldi, D. M., Chamberlain, P., Fetrow, & Wilson, J. E. (1997). Conducting ecology valid prevention research: Recruiting and retraining a "whole village" in multimethod, multiagent studies. *American Journal of Community Psychology, 25*(4), 471–492).

Capaldi, D. M., Crosby, L., & Stoolmiller, M. (1996). Predicting the timing of first sexual intercourse for at-risk adolescent males. *Child Development, 67,* 344–359.

Capaldi, D., & Patterson, G. R. (1991). The relation of parental transitions to boys' adjustment problems: I. A test of linear hypothesis. II. Mothers at risk for transitions and unskilled parenting. *Development and Psychopathology, 3,* 277–300.

Chamberlain, P. (1994). *Family connections: Treatment foster care for adolescents with delinquency.* Eugene, OR: Castalia.

Chamberlain, P., Patterson, G. R., Reid, J., & Kavanagh, K. (1984). Observation of client resistance. *Behavior Therapy, 15,* 144–155.

Chamberlain, P., & Reid, J. B. (1987). Parent observation and report of child symptoms. *Behavioral Assessment, 9,* 97–109.

Chamberlain, P., & Reid, J. B. (1998). Comparison of two community alternatives to incarceration for chronic juvenile offenders. *Journal of Consulting and Clinical Psychology, 6,* 624–633.

Chase-Lansdale, P. L., Brooks-Gunn, J., & Zamsky, E. S. (1994). Young African-

American multigenerational families in poverty: Quality of mothering and grandmothering. *Child Development, 65*(2), 373–393.

Chassin, L., Presson, C. C., & Sherman, S. J. (1990). Social psychological contributions to the understanding and prevention of adolescent cigarette smoking. *Personality and Social Psychology Bulletin, 16*, 133–151.

Chassin, L., Presson, C. C., Sherman, S. J., Montello, D., & McGrew, J. (1986). Changes in peer and parent influence during adolescence: Longitudinal versus cross-sectional perspectives on smoking initiation. *Developmental Psychology, 22*, 327–334.

Chilcoat, H. D., & Breslau, N. (1999). Pathways from ADHD to early drug use. *Journal of the American Academy of Child and Adolescent Psychiatry, 38*, 1347–1354.

Christensen, A., & Jacobson, N. S. (1994). Who (or what) can do psychotherapy: The status and challenge of nonprofessional therapies. *Psychological Science, 5*, 8–14.

Coatsworth, J. D., Szapocznik, J., Kurtines, W., & Santisteban, D. A. (1997). Culturally competent psychosocial interventions with antisocial problem behavior in Hispanic youth. In D. M. Stoff, J. Breiling, & J. D. Maser (Eds.), *Handbook of antisocial behavior* (pp. 103–114). New York: Wiley.

Coie, J. D., Dodge, K. A., & Coppotelli, H. (1982). Dimensions and types of social status: A cross-age perspective. *Developmental Psychology, 18*, 557–570.

Conger, R. D., Conger, K. J., Elder, G. H., Jr., Lorenz, F. O., Simons, R. L., & Whitbeck, L. B. (1992). A family process model of economic hardship and adjustment of early adolescent boys. *Child Development, 63*, 526–541.

Cook, T. D., & Campbell, D. T. (1979). *Quasi-experimentation: Design and analysis issues for field settings.* Boston: Houghton Mifflin.

Crick, N. R. (1996). The role of overt aggression, relational aggression, and prosocial behavior and the prediction of children's future social adjustment. *Child Development, 67*(5), 2317–2327.

Cronbach, L. J., & Glesar, G. C. (1965). *Psychological tests and personnel decisions.* Urbana: University of Illinois Press.

Dadds, M. R., Spence, S. H., Holland, D. E., Barrett, P. M., & Lacrens, K. R. (1997). Prevention and early intervention for anxiety disorders: A controlled trial. *Journal of Consulting and Clinical Psychology, 65*, 627–635.

Dawes, M. A., Dorn, L. D., Moss, H. B., Yao, J. K., Kirisci, L., Ammerman, R. T., & Tarter, R. E. (1999). Hormonal and behavioral homeostasis in boys at risk for substance abuse. *Drug and Alcohol Dependence, 55*, 165–176.

Dawes, R. M. (1994). *House of cards: Psychology and psychotherapy built on myth.* New York: Free Press.

Dawes, R. M., & Corrigan, B. (1974). Linear models in decision-making. *Psychological Bulletin, 81*, 95–106.

Dionne, R. (1997). *Indian family wellness intervention.* Unpublished manuscript. (Available from Child and Family Center, 195 West 12th Avenue, Eugene, OR 97401–3408.)

Dishion, T. J. (1998). *Advances in family-based interventions to adolescent drug abuse prevention.* Washington, DC: National Institute on Drug Abuse.

Dishion, T. J. (2000). Cross-setting consistency in early adolescent psychopathology: Deviant friendships and problem behavior sequelae. *Journal of Personality, 68*(6), 1109–1126.

Dishion, T. J., & Andrews, D. W. (1995). Preventing escalation in problem behaviors with high-risk young adolescents: Immediate and 1-year outcomes. *Journal of Consulting and Clinical Psychology, 63,* 538–548.

Dishion, T. J., Andrews, D. W., Kavanagh, K., & Soberman, L. H. (1996). Preventive interventions for high-risk youth: The Adolescent Transitions Program. In B. McMahon & R. D. Peters (Eds.), *Conduct disorders, substance abuse and delinquency: Prevention and early intervention approaches* (pp. 184–214). Newbury Park, CA: Sage.

Dishion, T. J., & Bullock, B. (2001). Parenting and adolescent problem behavior: An ecological analysis of the nurturance hypothesis. In J. G. Borkowski, S. Ramey, & M. Bristol-Power (Eds.), *Parenting and the child's world: Influences on intellectual, academic, and social-emotional development* (pp. 231–249). Mahwah, NJ: Erlbaum.

Dishion, T. J., Bullock, B. M., & Granic, I. (2002). Pragmatism in modeling peer influence: Dynamics, outcomes, and change processes. In D. Cicchetti & S. Hinshaw (Eds.), How prevention intervention studies in the field of developmental psychopathology can inform development theories and models [Special Issue]. *Development and Psychopathology, 14*(4), 995–1009.

Dishion, T. J., Bullock, B. M., & Owen, L. D. (2003). *Middle childhood parenting and early adolescent deviant friendship process.* Manuscript submitted for publication.

Dishion, T. J., Burraston, B., & Li, F. (2002). A multimethod and multitrait analysis of family management practices: Convergent and predictive validity. In W. Bukoski & Z. Amsel (Eds.), *Handbook for drug abuse prevention theory, science, and practice* (pp. 587–607). New York: Plenum Press.

Dishion, T. J., Capaldi, D., Spracklen, K. M., & Li, F. (1995). Peer ecology of male adolescent drug use. *Development and Psychopathology, 7,* 803–824.

Dishion, T. J., Capaldi, D. M., & Yoerger, K. (1999). Middle childhood antecedents to progression in male adolescent substance use: An ecological analysis of risk and protection. *Journal of Adolescent Research, 14,* 175–206.

Dishion, T. J., Duncan, T. E., Eddy, J. M., Fagot, B. I., & Fetrow, R. A. (1994). The world of parents and peers: Coercive exchanges and children's social adaption. *Social Development, 3,* 255–268.

Dishion, T. J., Eddy, J. M., Haas, E., Li, F., & Spracklen, K. (1997). Friendships and violent behavior during adolescence. *Social Development, 6,* 207–223.

Dishion, T. J., French, D. C., & Patterson, G. R. (1995). The development and ecology of antisocial behavior. In D. Cicchetti & D. J. Cohen (Eds.), *Developmental psychopathology: Vol. 2. Risk, disorder, and adaptation* (pp. 421–471). New York: Wiley.

Dishion, T. J., Gardner, K., Patterson, G. R., Reid, J. B., & Thibodeaux, S. (1983). *The Family Process Code: A multidimensional system for observing family interaction.* Unpublished coding manual. (Available from Oregon Social Learning Center, 160 East 4th Avenue, Eugene, OR 97401-2426.)

Dishion, T. J., & Kavanagh, K. (2002). The Adolescent Transitions Program: A family-centered prevention strategy for schools. In J. B. Reid, J. J. Snyder, & G. R. Patterson (Eds.), *The Oregon model: Understanding and altering the delinquency trajectory* (pp. 257–272). Washington, DC: American Psychological Association.

Dishion, T. J., Kavanagh, K., & Christianson, S. (1995). *Parenting in the teenage years.* (Video available from InterVision, 261 East 12th Avenue, Eugene, OR 97401 or 800-678-3455.)

Dishion, T. J., Kavanagh, K., Schneiger, A., Nelson, S., & Kaufman, N. (2002). Preventing early adolescent substance use: A family-centered strategy for the public middle-school ecology. In R. L. Spoth, K. Kavanagh, & T. J. Dishion (Eds.), Universal family-centered prevention strategies: Current findings and critical issues for public health impact [Special Issue]. *Prevention Science, 3,* 191–201.

Dishion, T. J., Kavanagh, K., Veltman, M., McCartney, T., Soberman, L., & Stormshak, E. A. (2003). *Family Management Curriculum V.20: Leader's guide.* Eugene, OR: Child and Family Center Publications (*http://cfc. uoregon.edu*).

Dishion, T. J., & Loeber, R. (1985). Male adolescent marijuana and alcohol use: The role of parents and peers revisited. *American Journal of Drug and Alcohol Abuse, 11,* 11–25.

Dishion, T. J., Loeber, R., Stouthamer-Loeber, M., & Patterson, G. R. (1984). Skill deficits and male adolescent delinquency. *Journal of Abnormal Child Psychology, 12,* 37–54.

Dishion, T. J., McCord, J., & Poulin, F. (1999). When interventions harm: Peer groups and problem behavior. *American Psychologist, 54,* 1–10.

Dishion, T. J., & McMahon, R. J. (1998). Parental monitoring and the prevention of child and adolescent problem behavior: A conceptual and empirical formulation. *Clinical Child and Family Psychology Review, 1,* 61–75.

Dishion, T. J., Moore, K. J., Prescott, A. & Kavanagh, K. (1989). *Teen Focus: A behavior change curriculum for young adolescents* [Videotape]. (Available from InterVision, 261 East 12th Avenue, Suite 100, Eugene, OR 97401.)

Dishion, T. J., & Owen, L. D. (2002). A longitudinal analysis of friendships and substance use: Bi-directional influence from adolescence to adulthood. *Developmental Psychology, 38*(4), 480–491.

Dishion, T. J., & Patterson, G. R. (1992). Age effects in parent training outcome. *Behavior Therapy, 23,* 719–729.

Dishion, T. J., & Patterson, G. R. (1993). Antisocial behavior: Using a multiple gating strategy. In M. I. Singer, L. T. Singer, & T. M. Anglin (Eds.), *Handbook for screening adolescents at psychosocial risk* (pp. 375–399). New York: Lexington.

Dishion, T. J., & Patterson, G. R. (1997). The timing and severity of antisocial behavior: Three hypotheses within an ecological framework. In D. Stoff, J. Brieling, & J. Maser (Eds.), *Handbook of antisocial behavior* (pp. 205–217). New York: Wiley.

Dishion, T. J., & Patterson, G. R. (1999). Model-building in developmental psychopathology: A pragmatic approach to understanding and intervention. *Journal of Clinical Child Psychology, 28,* 502–512.

Dishion, T. J., Patterson, G. R., & Kavanagh, K. (1992). An experimental test of the coercion model: Linking theory, measurement, and intervention. In J. McCord & R. E. Tremblay (Eds.), *The interaction of theory and practice: Experimental studies of interventions* (pp. 253–282). New York: Guilford Press.

Dishion, T. J., Patterson, G. R., Stoolmiller, M., & Skinner, M. (1991). Family, school, and behavioral antecedents to early adolescent involvement with antisocial peers. *Developmental Psychology, 27,* 172–180.

Dishion, T. J., Poulin, F., & Medici Skaggs, N. (2000). The ecology of premature autonomy in adolescence: Biological and social influences. In K. A. Kerns, J. M. Contreras, & A. M. Neal-Barnett (Eds.), *Family and peers: Linking two social worlds* (pp. 27–45). Westport, CT: Praeger.

Dishion, T. J., Reid, J. B., & Patterson, G. R. (1988). Empirical guidelines for a family intervention for adolescent drug use. *Journal of Chemical Dependency Treatment, 1,* 189–222.

Dishion, T. J., Rivera, E. K., Jones, L., Verberkmoes, S., & Patras, J. (2002). *Relationship Process Code.* Unpublished coding manual. (Available from Child and Family Center, University of Oregon, 195 West 12th Avenue, Eugene, OR 97401–3408.)

Dishion, T. J., Spracklen, K. M., Andrews, D. M., & Patterson, G. R. (1996). Deviancy training in male adolescent friendships. *Behavior Therapy, 27*(1), 373–390.

Dishion, T. J., & Stormshak, E. (in press). *An ecological approach to child clinical and counseling psychology.* Washington, DC: APA Books.

Dodge, K. A. (1991). The structure and function of proactive and reactive aggression. In D. J. Pepler & K. H. Rubin (Eds.), *The development and treatment of childhood aggression* (pp. 201–218). Hillsdale, NJ: Erlbaum.

Dodge, K. A. (1993). The future of research and the treatment of conduct disorder. *Development and Psychopathology, 5,* 311–319.

Dodge, K. A., & Coie, J. D. (1987). Social-information-processing factors in reactive and proactive aggression in children's peer groups. *Journal of Personality and Social Psychology, 53,* 1146–1158.

Donovan, J. E., Jessor, R., & Costa, F. M. (1993). Structure of health-enhancing behavior in adolescents: A latent-variable approach. *Journal of Health and Social Behavior, 34,* 346–362.

Dumas, J. E. (1989). Treating antisocial behavior in children: Child and family approaches. *Clinical Psychology Review, 9,* 197–222.

Duncan, O. D., Ohlin, L. E., Reiss, A. J., & Stanton, H. R. (1953). Formal devices for making selection decisions. *American Journal of Sociology, 58,* 573–584.

Duran, E., & Duran, B. (1995). *Native American postcolonial psychology.* Albany: State University of New York Press.

Dwyer, J. H. (1983). *Statistical models for the social and behavior sciences.* New York: Oxford University Press.

Eccles, J. S., Lord, S. E., & Roeser, R. W. (1995). Round holes, square pegs, rocky roads, and sore feet: The impact of stage–environment fit on young adolescents' experiences in schools and families. In D. Cicchetti & S. Toth (Eds.), *Rochester Symposium on Developmental Psychopathology: Vol. 7:*

Adolescence: Opportunities and challenges (pp. 47–92). Rochester, NY: University of Rochester Press.

Eccles, J. S., Midgley, C., Wigfield, A., Buchanan, C. M., Reuman, D., Flanagan, C., & MacIver, D. (1993). Development during adolescence: The impact of stage–environment fit on adolescents' experience in schools and families. *American Psychologist, 48*, 90–101.

Eddy, J. M., Dishion, T. J., & Stoolmiller, M. (1998). The analysis of change in children and families: Methodological and conceptual issues embedded in intervention studies. *Journal of Abnormal Child Psychology, 26*, 53–69.

Egeland, B., & Susman-Stillman, A. (1996). Dissociation as a mediator of child abuse across generations. *Child Abuse and Neglect, 20*, 1123–1132.

Eisenberg, N., Carlo, G., Murphy, B., & Van Court, P. (1995). Prosocial development in late adolescence: A longitudinal study. *Child Development, 66*, 1179–1197.

Elder, G. H., Van Nguyen, T., & Caspi, A. (1985). Linking family hardship to children's lives. *Child Development, 56*, 361–375.

Elliott, D. S., & Voss, H. L. (1974). *Delinquency and dropout.* Lexington, MA: Lexington.

Farrington, D. P. (1991). Childhood aggression and adult violence: Early precursors and later life outcomes. In D. J. Pepler & K. H. Rubin (Eds.), *The development and treatment of childhood aggression* (pp. 5–30). Hillsdale, NJ: Erlbaum.

Fergusson, D. M., & Horwood, L. J. (2002). Male and female offending trajectories. *Development and Psychopathology, 14*, 159–177.

Fisher, P. A., & Ball, T. J. (2002). The Indian Family Wellness Project: An application of the Tribal Participatory Research model. In R. L. Spoth, K. Kavanagh, & T. J. Dishion (Eds.), Universal family-centered prevention strategies: Current findings and critical issues for public health impact [Special Issue]. *Prevention Science, 3*, 235–240.

Fisher, P. A., Fagot, B. I., & Leve, C. S. (1998). Assessment of family stress across low-, medium-, and high-risk samples using the family events checklist. *Family Relations, 47*, 1–5.

Fleischman, M. (1979). Using parenting salaries to control attrition and cooperation in therapy. *Behavior Therapy, 10*, 111–116.

Fogel, B. S. (1996). A neuropsychiatric approach to impairment of goal-directed behavior. *American Psychiatric Press Review of Psychiatry, 15*, 163–173.

Forgatch, M. S. (1989). Patterns and outcome in family problem solving: The disrupting effect of negative emotion. *Journal of Marriage and Family, 51*, 115–124.

Forgatch, M. (1991). The clinical science vortex: Developing a theory for antisocial behavior. In D. Pepler (Ed.), *The development and treatment of childhood aggression* (pp. 291–315). Hillsdale, NJ: Erlbaum.

Forgatch, M. S., Fetrow, B., & Lathrop, M. (1985). *Solving problems in family interactions.* Unpublished training manual. (Available from Oregon Social Learning Center, 160 East 4th Avenue, Eugene, OR 97401-2426.)

Forgatch, M. S., & Patterson, G. R. (1989). *Parents and adolescents living together: II. Family problem-solving.* Eugene, OR: Castalia.

Forgatch, M. S., Patterson, G. R., & Skinner, M. L. (1988). A mediational model for the effect of divorce on antisocial behavior in boys. In E. M. Hethering-ton & J. D. Aresteh (Eds.), *Impact of divorce, single parenting, and step-parenting on children* (pp. 135–154). Hillsdale, NJ: Erlbaum.

Forgatch, M. S., & Stoolmiller, M. (1994). Emotions as contexts for adolescent delinquency. *Journal of Research on Adolescence, 4,* 601–614.

Friedman, A. S. (1989). Family therapy versus parent groups: Effects on adolescent drug abusers. *American Journal of Family Therapy, 17,* 335–347.

French, D. C., & Weih, S. (1990). *House rules: A measure of parental monitoring.* Unpublished manuscript.

Gardner, F. E. M. (1992). Parent–child interaction and conduct disorders. *Educational Psychology Review, 4,* 135–163.

Gorman-Smith, D., & Tolan, P. (1998). The role of exposure to community violence and developmental problems among inner city youth. *Development and Psychopathology, 10,* 101–116.

Gottfredson, D. (1988). An evaluation of an organization development approach to reducing school disorder. *Evaluation Review, 11,* 739–763.

Gottman, J. M. (1979). *Marital interaction: Experimental investigations.* New York: Academic Press.

Gottman, J. M. (1998). Psychology and the study of marital process. *Annual Review of Psychology, 49,* 169–197.

Gottman, J. M., & Levenson, R. W. (1986). Assessing the role of emotion in marriage. *Behavioral Assessment, 8,* 31–48.

Granic, I., Dishion, T. J., & Hollenstein, T. (2003). The family ecology of adolescence: A dynamic systems perspective on normative development. In G. R. Adams & M. Berzonsky (Eds.), *The Blackwell handbook of adolescence* (pp. 60–91). Oxford, UK: Blackwell.

Granic, I., & Lamey, A. V. (2002). Combining dynamic systems and multivariate analyses to compare the mother–child interactions of externalizing subtypes. *Journal of Abnormal Child Psychology, 30,* 265–283.

Grotpeter, J. K., & Crick, N. R. (1996). Relational aggression, overt aggression, and friendship. *Child Development, 67,* 123–150.

Harris, J. R. (1995). Where is the child's environment?: A group socialization theory of development. *Psychological Review, 102,* 458–489.

Hawkins, J. D., Catalano, R. F., & Miller, J. Y. (1992). Risk and protective factors for alcohol and other drug problems in adolescence and early adulthood: Implications for substance abuse prevention. *Psychological Bulletin, 112,* 64–105.

Hawkins, D. L., Pepler, D. J., & Craig, W. M. (2001). Naturalistic observations of peer interventions in bullying. *Social Development, 10*(4), 512–527.

Henggeler, S. W., Melton, G. B., & Smith, L. A. (1992). Family preservation using multisystemic treatment: An effective alternative to incarcerating serious juvenile offenders. *Journal of Consulting and Clinical Psychology, 60,* 953–961.

Henggeler, S. W., Rodnick, J. D., Borduin, C. M., Hanson, C. L., Watson, S. M., & Urey, J. R. (1986). Multisystemic treatment of juvenile offenders: Effects on adolescent behavior and family interaction. *Developmental Psychology, 22,* 132–141.

Henggeler, S. W., Schoenwald, S. K., Borduin, C. M., Rowland, M. D., &

Cunningham, P. B. (1998). *Multisystemic treatment of antisocial behavior in children and adolescents.* New York: Guilford Press.

Hernstein, R. J. (1961). Relative and absolute strength of response as a function of frequency of reinforcement. *Journal of Experimental Analysis of Behavior, 4,* 267–272.

Higgins, S. T., Budney, A. J., Bickel, W. K., Hughes, J. R., Foerg, F., & Badger, G. (1993). Achieving cocaine abstinence with a behavioral approach. *American Journal of Psychiatry, 150,* 763–769.

Hinshaw, S. P. (1987). On the distinction between attentional deficits/hyperactivity and conduct problems/aggression in child psychopathology. *Psychological Bulletin, 101,* 443–463.

Hoagwood, K., & Koretz, D. (1996). Embedding prevention services within systems of care: Strengthening the nexus for children. *Applied and Prevention Psychology, 5,* 225–234.

Hogansen, J., & Dishion, T. J. (2001, June). *Promoting change in parent group interventions for adolescent problem behavior.* Poster presented at the 10th Scientific Meeting of the International Society for Research in Child and Adolescent Psychopathology, Vancouver, BC, Canada.

Holmes, T. H., & Rahe, R. H. (1967). The social readjustment rating scale. *Journal of Psychosomatic Research, 11,* 213–218.

Hops, H., Sherman, L., & Biglan, A. (1990). Maternal depression, marital discord, and children's behavior: A developmental perspective. In G. R. Patterson (Ed.), *Depression and aggression in family interaction* (pp. 185–308). Hillsdale, NJ: Erlbaum.

Horner, R. H., Day, H. M., & Day, J. R. (1997). Using neuralized routines to reduce problem behavior. *Journal of Applied Behavior Analysis, 30,* 601–614.

Huey, S. J., Henggeler, S. W., Brondino, M. J., & Pickrel, S. G. (2000). Mechanisms of change in multisystemic therapy: Reducing delinquent behavior through therapist adherence and improved family and peer functioning. *Journal of Clinical Child Psychology, 68,* 451–467.

Huston, T. L., & Vangelisti, A. L. (1991). Socioemotional behavior and satisfaction in marital relationships: A longitudinal study. *Journal of Personality and Social Psychology, 61,* 721–733.

Irvine, A. B., Biglan, A., Metzler, C. W., Smolkowski, K., & Ary, D. V. (1999). The effectiveness of a parenting skills program for parents of middle school students in small communities. *Journal of Consulting and Clinical Psychology, 67,* 811–825.

Izard, C. E., & Harris, P. (1995). Emotional development and developmental psychopathology. In D. Cicchetti & D. J. Cohen (Eds.), *Developmental psychopathology: Vol. 2. Risk, disorder, and adaptation* (pp. 467–503). New York: Wiley.

Jacobsen, N. S., & Truax, P. (1991). Clinical significance: A statistical approach to defining meaningful change in psychotherapy research. *Journal of Consulting and Clinical Psychology, 59,* 12–19.

Jessor, R., & Jessor, S. L. (1977). *Problem behavior and psychosocial development.* New York: Academic Press.

Johnson, S. M., & Christensen, A. (1975). Multiple criteria follow-up of behavior modification. *Journal of Abnormal Child Psychology, 3,* 135–154.

Johnson, C. A., Pentz, M. A., Weber, M. D., Dwyer, J. H., MacKinnan, D. P., Flay, B. R., Baer, N. A., & Hansen, W. B. (1990). The relative effectiveness of comprehensive community programming for drug abuse prevention with risk and low risk adolescents. *Journal of Consulting and Clinical Psychology, 58,* 447–456.

Kandel, D. B., Davies, M., Karus, D., & Yamaguchi, K. (1986). The consequences in young adulthood of adolescent drug involvement. *Archives of General Psychiatry, 43,* 746–754.

Kavanagh, K., Burraston, B., Dishion, T. J., & Schneiger, A. (2000, March). *Identification of middle school students' risk behavior: Contextual influences of gender and ethnicity.* Poster presented at the Eighth Biennial Meeting of the Society for Research on Adolescence, Chicago, IL.

Kavanagh, K., Dishion, T. J., Winter, C., & Burraston, B. (2000, June). *Processes of family and school engagement: Adolescent Transitions Program.* Paper presented at the Eighth Annual Meeting of the Society for Prevention Research, Montreal, Quebec, Canada.

Kavanagh, K., & Hops, H. (1994). Good girls? Bad boys?: Gender and development as contexts for diagnosis and treatment. In T. H. Ollendick & R. J. Prinz (Eds.), *Advances in clinical child psychology* (Vol. 16, pp. 45–69). New York: Plenum Press.

Kazdin, A. E. (1993). Treatment of conduct disorder: Progress and directions in psychotherapy research. *Development and Psychopathology, 5,* 277–310.

Kazdin, A. E. (2002). Psychosocial treatments for conduct disorder in children and adolescents. In P. Nathan & J. Gorman (Eds.), *A guide to treatments that work* (2nd ed., pp. 57–85). London: Oxford University Press.

Kazdin, A. E., Siegel, T. C., & Bass, D. (1992). Cognitive problem solving skills training and parent management training in the treatment of antisocial behavior in children. *Journal of Consulting and Clinical Psychology, 60,* 733–747.

Kazdin, A. E., & Weisz, J. R. (1998). Identifying and developing empirically supported child and adolescent treatments. *Journal of Consulting and Clinical Psychology, 66,* 19–36.

Kellam, S. G. (1990). Developmental epidemiological framework for family research on depression and aggression. In G. R. Patterson (Ed.), *Depression and aggression in family interaction* (pp. 11–48). Hillsdale, NJ: Erlbaum.

Kellam, S. G., Brown, C. H., Rubin, B. R., & Ensminger, M. E. (1983). Paths leading to teenage psychiatric symptoms and substance use: Developmental epidemiological studies in Woodlawn. In S. R. Guze, F. J. Earns, & J. E. Barrett (Eds.), *Childhood psychopathology and development* (pp. 17–51). New York: Raven Press.

Kelly, J. G. (1988). *A guide to conducting preventive research in the community: First steps.* New York: Haworth.

Kochanska, G. (1993). Toward a synthesis of parental socialization and child temperament in early development of conscience. *Child Development, 64,* 325–347.

Kumpfer, K. L., Alvarado, R., Smith, P., & Bellamy, N. (2002). Cultural sensitivity and adaptation in family-based prevention interventions. In R. L. Spoth, K. Kavanagh, & T. J. Dishion (Eds.), Universal family-centered prevention strategies: Current findings and critical issues for public health impact [Special Issue]. *Prevention Science, 3,* 241–246.

Kumpfer, K. L., Molgaard, V., & Spoth, R. (1996). The strengthening families program for the prevention of delinquency and drug abuse. In R. D. Peters & R. J. McMahon (Eds.), *Preventing childhood disorders, substance abuse, and delinquency* (pp. 241–267). Newbury, CA: Sage.

Landman, J. T., & Dawes, R. M. (1982). Psychotherapy outcome: Smith and Glass' conclusions stand up under scrutiny. *American Psychologist, 37*(5), 504–516.

Lewinsohn, P. M., & Clark, G. N. (1990). Cognitive-behavioral treatment for depressed adolescents. *Behavior Therapy, 19,* 385–401.

Lewis, M. D. (2000). The promise of dynamic systems approaches for an integrated account of human development. *Child Development, 71,* 36–43.

Lewis, R. A., Piercy, F. P., Sprendle, D. H., & Trepper, T. J. (1990). Family-based interventions for helping drug-using adolescents. *Journal of Adolescent Research, 5,* 82–95.

Liddle, H. A. (1999). Theory in a family-based therapy for adolescent drug abuse. *Journal of Clinical Child Psychology, 28,* 521–532.

Linehan, M. M. (1987). Dialectical behavior therapy for borderline personality disorder. *Bulletin of the Menninger Clinic, 51,* 261–276.

Lipsey, M. W. (1992). Juvenile delinquency treatment: A meta-analytic inquiry into the variability of effects. In T. D. Cook, H. Cooper, D. S. Cordray, H. Hartmann, L. V. Hedges, R. J. Light, T. A. Lewis, & F. Mosteller (Eds.), *Meta-analysis for explanation: A casebook* (pp. 83–125). New York: Russell Sage Foundation.

Lochman, J. E., Burch, P. R., Curry, J. F., & Lampron, L. B. (1984). Treatment and generalization effects of cognitive behavioral and goal-setting interventions with aggressive boys. *Journal of Consulting and Clinical Psychology, 52,* 915–916.

Lochman, J. E., & Wells, K. C. (1996). A social-cognitive intervention with aggressive children: Prevention effects and contextual implementation issues. In R. D. Peters & R. J. McMahon (Eds.), *Preventing childhood disorders, substance abuse, and delinquency* (pp. 111–143). Thousand Oaks, CA: Sage.

Lochman, J. E., White, K. J., Curry, J. F., & Rumer, R. R. (1992). Antisocial behavior. In V. B. Van Hasselt & D. J. Kolko (Eds.), *Inpatient behavior therapy for children and adolescents* (pp. 277–312). New York: Plenum Press.

Loeber, R. (1982). The stability of antisocial and delinquent child behavior: A review. *Child Development, 53*(6), 1431–1446.

Loeber, R. (1988). Natural histories of conduct problems, delinquency, and associated substance use: Evidence for developmental progressions. In B. B. Lahey & A. E. Casdin (Eds.), *Advances in clinical child psychopathology* (Vol. 2, pp. 73–124). New York: Plenum Press.

Loeber, R., & Dishion, T. J. (1983). Early predictors of male delinquency: A review. *Psychological Bulletin, 94*, 68–99.

Loeber, R., & Dishion, T. J. (1987). Antisocial and delinquent youth: Methods for their early identification. In J. D. Burchard & S. N. Burchard (Eds.), *Prevention of delinquent behavior* (Vol. 10, pp. 75–89). Newbury Park, CA: Sage.

Loeber, R., Dishion, T. J., & Patterson, G. R. (1984). Multiple gating: A multistage assessment procedure for identifying youths at risk for delinquency. *Journal of Research in Crime and Delinquency, 21*, 7–32.

Loeber, R., & Schmaling, K. B. (1985). The utility of differentiating between mixed and pure forms of antisocial child behavior. *Journal of Abnormal Child Psychology, 13*, 315–336.

Maccoby, E. (1992). The role of parents in the socialization of children: An historical overview. *Developmental Psychology, 28*, 1006–1017.

Maccoby, E. E., Depner, C. E., & Mnookin, R. H. (1990). Co-parenting in the second year after divorce. *Journal of Marriage and the Family, 52*, 141–155.

Magnusson, D. (1988). Aggressive, hyperactivity, and autonomic activity/reactivity in the development of social maladjustment. In D. Magnusson (Ed.), *Paths through life: Individual development from an interactional perspective: A longitudinal study* (Vol. 1, pp. 153–175). Hillsdale, NJ: Erlbaum.

McCord, J. (1978). A third-year follow-up of treatment effects. *American Psychologist, 37*, 1477–1486.

McCord, J. (1979). Some child-rearing antecedents of criminal behavior in adult men. *Journal of Personality and Social Psychology, 37*, 1477–1486.

McCord, J. (1981). Consideration of some effects of a counseling program. In S. E. Martin, L. B. Sechrest, & R. Redner (Eds.), *New directions in the rehabilitation of criminal offenders* (pp. 394–405). Washington, DC: National Academy of Sciences.

McCord, J. (1992). The Cambridge–Somerville Study: A pioneering longitudinal–experimental study of delinquency prevention. In J. McCord & R. E. Tremblay (Eds.), *Preventing antisocial behavior: Interventions from birth through adolescence* (pp. 196–206). New York: Guilford Press.

McCord, J. (1997, April). *Some unanticipated consequences of summer camps.* Paper presented at the Biennial Meeting of the Society for Research in Child Development, Washington, DC.

McDowell, J. J. (1988). Matching theory in natural human environments. *Behavior Analyst, 11*, 95–109.

McLoyd, V. C. (1990). The impact of economic hardship on Black families and children: Psychological distress, parenting, and socioemotional development. *Child Development, 61*, 311–346.

McMahon, R. J., Tiedemann, G. L., Forehand, R., & Griest, D. L. (1993). Parental satisfaction with parent training to modify child noncompliance. *Behavior Therapy, 15*, 295–303.

Meehl, P. E. (1978). Theoretical risks and tabular asterisks: Sir Karl, Sir Ronald, and the slow progress of soft psychology. *Journal of Consulting and Clinical Psychology, 46*, 806–834.

Meehl, P. E., & Rosen, A. (1955). Antecedent probability and the efficiency of psychometric signs, patterns, or cutting scores. *Psychological Bulletin, 52,* 194–216.

Metzler, C. W., Biglan, A., Rusby, J. C., & Sprague, J. R. (2001). Evaluation of a comprehensive behavior management program to improve school-wide positive behavior support. *Education and Treatment of Children, 24,* 448–479.

Metzler, C. W., Noell, J., & Biglan, A. (1992). The validation of a construct of high-risk sexual behavior in heterosexual adolescents. *Journal of Adolescent Research, 7,* 233–249.

Miller, W. R. (1987). Motivation and treatment goals. *Drugs and Society, 1,* 133–151.

Miller, W. R. (1989). Increasing motivation for change. In R. K. Hester & W. R. Miller (Eds.), *Handbook of alcoholism treatment approaches: Effective alternatives* (pp. 67–80). Elmsford, NY: Pergamon.

Miller, W. R., Benefield, R. G., & Tonigan, J. S. (2001). Enhancing motivation for change in problem drinking: A controlled comparison of two therapist styles. In C. E. Hill (Ed.), *Helping skills: The empirical foundation* (pp. 243–255). Washington, DC: American Psychological Association.

Miller, W. R., & Brown, J. M. (1991). Self-regulation as a conceptual basis for the prevention and treatment of addictive behaviors. In N. Heather, W. R. Miller, & J. Greeley (Eds.), *Self-control and addictive behaviours* (pp. 3–82). Sydney, Australia: Maxwell MacMillan.

Miller, W. R., & Rollnick, S. (2002). *Motivational interviewing: Preparing people for change* (2nd ed.). New York: Guilford Press.

Miller, W. R., & Sovereign, R. G. (1989). The checkup: A model for early intervention in addictive behaviors. In T. Loberg, W. R. Miller, P. E. Nathan, & G. A. Marlatt (Eds.), *Addictive behaviors: Prevention and early intervention* (pp. 219–231). Amsterdam: Swets & Zeitlinger.

Minkin, N., Braukman, C. J., Minkin, B. J., Timbers, G. D., Timbers, B. J., Fixsen, D. L., Phillips, E. L., & Wolf, M. M. (1976). The social validation and training of conversational skills. *Journal of Applied Behavior Analysis, 9,* 127–139.

Minuchin, S., & Fishman, H. C. (1981). *Family therapy techniques.* Cambridge, MA: Harvard University Press.

Moffitt, T. E. (1993). Adolescence-limited and life course persistent antisocial behavior: Developmental taxonomy. *Psychological Review, 100,* 674–701.

Moffitt, T. E., Caspi, A., Rutter, M., & Silva, P. A. (2001). *Sex differences in antisocial behaviour: Conduct disorder, delinquency, and violence in the Dunedin Longitudinal Study.* New York: Cambridge University Press.

Moore, K. J., Osgood, W. D., Larzelere, R. E., & Chamberlain, P. (1994). Use of pooled time series in the study of naturally occurring clinical events and problem behavior in a foster care setting. *Journal of Consulting and Clinical Psychology, 62,* 718–728.

Morrill, W. H., Oetting, E. R., & Hurst, J. C. (1974). Dimensions of counselor functioning. *Personnel and Guidance Journal, 52*(6), 354–359.

Mrazek, P. J., & Haggerty, R. J. (1995). *Reducing risks for mental disorders: Frontiers for preventive intervention research.* Washington, DC: National Academy Press.

Newcomb, M., & Bentler, P. (1988). *Consequences of adolescent drug use.* Newbury Park, CA: Sage.

O'Dell, S. L. (1982) Enhancing parent involvement training: A discussion. *Behavior Therapist, 5*(1), 9–13.

Olds, D. L. (2002). Prenatal and infancy home visiting by nurses: From randomized trials to community replication. In R. L. Spoth, K. Kavanagh, & T. J. Dishion (Eds.), Universal family-centered prevention strategies: Current findings and critical issues for public health impact [Special Issue]. *Prevention Science, 3,* 153–172.

O'Leary, S. G. (1995). Parental discipline mistakes. *Current Directions in Psychological Science, 4,* 11–13.

Olweus, D. (1979). Stability of aggressive reaction patterns in males: A review. *Psychological Bulletin, 86,* 852–875.

Olweus, D. (1991). Bully/victim problems among school children: Basic facts and effects of a school based intervention program. In D. J. Pepler & K. H. Rubin (Eds.), *The development and treatment of childhood aggression* (pp. 411–448). Hillsdale, NJ: Erlbaum.

O'Malley, P. M., Bachman, J. G., & Johnston, L. D. (1988). Period, age, and cohort effects on substance use among young Americans: A decade of change, 1976–86. *American Journal of Public Health, 78*(10), 1315–1321.

Patterson, G. R. (1974). Interventions for boys with conduct problems: Multiple settings, treatments, and criteria. *Journal of Consulting and Clinical Psychology, 42,* 471–481.

Patterson, G. R. (1982). *A social learning approach: III. Coercive family process.* Eugene, OR: Castalia.

Patterson, G. R. (1993). Orderly change in a stable world: The antisocial trait as a chimera. *Journal of Consulting and Clinical Psychology, 61,* 911–919.

Patterson, G. R. (1997). Performance models for parenting: A social interactional perspective. In J. E. Grusec & L. Kuczynski (Eds.), *Parenting and children's internalization of values: A handbook of contemporary theory* (pp. 193–226). New York: Wiley.

Patterson, G. R., & Chamberlain, P. (1994). A functional analysis of resistance during parent training therapy. *Clinical Psychology: Science and Practice, 1,* 53–70.

Patterson, G. R., & Dishion, T. J. (1985) Contributions of families and peers to delinquency. *Criminology, 23,* 63–79.

Patterson, G. R., Dishion, T. J., & Chamberlain, P. (1993). Outcomes and methodological issues relating to treatment of antisocial children. In T. R. Giles (Ed.), *Effective psychotherapy: A handbook of comparative research* (pp. 43–88). New York: Plenum Press.

Patterson, G. R., & Forgatch, M. S. (1985). Therapist behavior as a determinant for client resistance: A paradox for the behavior modifier. *Journal of Consulting and Clinical Psychology, 53*(6), 846–851.

Patterson, G. R., & Forgatch, M. (1987). *Parents and adolescents living together: I. The basics.* Eugene, OR: Castalia.

Patterson, G. R., Reid, J. B., & Dishion, T. J. (1992). *A social learning approach: IV. Antisocial boys.* Eugene, OR: Castalia.

Patterson, G. R., Reid, J. B., Jones, R. R., & Conger, R. E. (1975). *A social learning approach to family intervention: Families with aggressive children* (Vol. 1). Eugene, OR: Castalia.

Paul, G. L., & Menditto, A. A. (1992). Affectiveness of inpatient treatment programs for mentally ill adults in public psychiatric facilities. *Applied and Preventative Psychology, 1,* 41–63.

Peery, C. J. (1979). Popular, amiable, isolated, rejected: A reconceptualization of sociometric status in preschool children. *Child Development, 50,* 1231–1234.

Pentz, M. A., MacKinnon, D. P., Dwyer, J. H., Wang, E. Y. J., Hansen, W. B., Flay, B. R., & Johnson, C. A. (1989). Longitudinal effects of the Midwestern Prevention Project on regular and experimental smoking in adolescents. *Preventive Medicine, 18,* 304–321.

Poulin, F., & Boivin, M. (2000). The role of proactive and reactive aggression in the formation and the development of friendships in boys. *Developmental Psychology, 36*(2), 233–240.

Poulin, F., Dishion, T. J., & Burraston, B. (2001). Three-year iatrogenic effects associated with aggregating high-risk adolescents in preventive interventions. *Applied Developmental Science, 5,* 214–224.

Prinz, R. J., Foster, S., Kent, R. N., & O'Leary, D. K. (1979). Multivariate assessment of conflict in distressed and nondistressed mother–adolescent dyads. *Journal of Applied Behavior Analysis, 12*(4), 691–700.

Prinz, R. J., & Miller, G. E. (1994). Family-based treatment for childhood antisocial behavior: Experimental influences on dropout and engagement. *Journal of Consulting and Clinical Psychology, 62,* 645–650.

Prochaska, J. O., & DiClemente, C. (1982). Transtheoretical therapy: Toward a more integrated model of change. *Psychotherapy: Theory, Research, and Practice, 19,* 276–288.

Prochaska, J. O., & DiClemente, C. C. (1986). Toward a comprehensive model of change. In W. Miller & N. Heather (Eds.), *Treating addictive behaviors: Processes of change* (pp. 3–27). New York: Plenum Press.

Prochaska, J. O., Velicer, W. F., Guadagnoli, E., & Rossi, J. S. (1991). Patterns of change: Dynamic typology applied to smoking cessation. *Multivariate Behavioral Research, 26,* 83–107.

Pulkkinen, L. (1982). The search for alternatives to aggression. In A. P. Goldstein & M. Segall (Eds.), *Aggression in global perspective* (pp. 104–144). New York: Pergamon.

Pulkkinen, L. (1996). Proactive and reactive aggression in early adolescence as precursors to anti- and prosocial behavior in young adults. *Aggressive Behavior, 22,* 241–257.

Pulkkinen, L., & Ronka, A. (1994). Personal control over development, identity formation, and future orientation as components of life orientation: A developmental approach. *Developmental Psychology, 30,* 260–271.

Radloff, L. S. (1977). The CES-D scale: A self-report depression scale for research in the general population. *Applied Psychological Measurement, 1,* 385–401.

Rao, S. A. (1998). *The short-term impact of the Family Check-Up: A brief moti-*

vational intervention for at-risk families. Unpublished doctoral dissertation, University of Oregon, Eugene.

Rescorla, R. A. (1987). A Pavlovian analysis of goal-directed behavior. *American Psychologist, 42,* 119–129.

Rhee, S. H., & Waldman, I. D. (2002). Genetic and environmental influences on antisocial behavior: A meta-analysis of twin and adoption studies. *Psychological Bulletin, 128,* 490–529.

Robin, A. L., & Foster, S. L. (1989). *Negotiating parent–adolescent conflict: A behavioral–family systems approach.* New York: Guilford Press.

Robins, L. N., & Przybeck, T. R. (1985). Age of onset of drug use as a factor in drug and other disorders. In C. L. Jones & R. J. Battjes (Eds.), *Etiology of drug abuse: Implications for prevention* (Research Monograph No. 56, pp. 178–193). Rockville, MD: National Institute on Drug Abuse.

Robins, M. S., Alexander, J. F., Newell, R. N., & Turner, C. W. (1996). The immediate effect of reframing on client attitude and family therapy. *Journal of Family Psychology, 10,* 28–34.

Rogers, C. R. (1940). The process of therapy. *Journal of Consulting Psychology, 4,* 161–164.

Rogers, C. R. (1957). The necessary and sufficient conditions of therapeutic personality change. *Journal of Consulting Psychology, 21,* 95–103.

Rosenbaum, E., & Kandel, D. B. (1990). Early onset of adolescent sexual behavior and drug involvement. *Journal of Marriage and the Family, 52,* 783–798.

Rothbart, M. K., & Bates, J. E. (1998). Temperament. In W. Damon (Series Ed.) & N. Eisenberg (Vol. Ed.), *Handbook of child psychology: Vol. 3. Social, emotional, and personality development* (5th ed., pp. 105–176). New York: Wiley.

Rothbart, M. K., Posner, M. I., & Hershey, K. L. (1995). Temperament, attention, and developmental psychopathology. In D. Cicchetti & D. J. Cohen (Eds.), *Developmental psychopathology: Vol. 1. Theory and methods* (pp. 315–340). New York: Wiley.

Rutter, M. (1985). Family and school influences on behavioural development. *Journal of Child Psychology and Psychiatry and Allied Disciplines, 26,* 349–368.

Rutter, M. (1989, April). *Peer relations and developmental psychopathology.* Paper presented at the preconference on Research on Peer Relations, Biennial Meeting for the Society for Research in Child Development, Kansas City, MO.

Sackett, G. P. (1979). The lag sequential analysis of contingency and cyclicity in behavioral interaction and research. In J. D. Osofsky (Ed.), *Handbook of infant development* (pp. 623–649). New York: Wiley.

Sanders, M. R., & Lawton, J. M. (1993). Discussing assessment findings with families: A guided participation model of information transfer. *Child and Family Behavior Therapy, 15,* 5–33.

Sanders, M. R., Turner, K. M. T., & Markie-Dadds, C. (2002). The development and dissemination of the Triple P-Positive Parenting Program: A multilevel, evidence-based system of parenting and family support. In R. L. Spoth, K.

Kavanagh, & T. J. Dishion (Eds.), Universal family-centered prevention strategies: Current findings and critical issues for public health impact [Special Issue]. *Prevention Science, 3,* 173–189.

Sarason, S. B. (1981). An asocial psychology and a misdirected clinical psychology. *American Psychologist, 36*(8), 827–836.

Schmidt, S. E., Liddle, H. A., & Dakof, G. A. (1996). Changes in parenting practices and adolescent drug abuse during multidimensional family therapy. *Journal of Family Psychology, 10,* 12–27.

Shaw, D. S., Owens, E. B., Vondra, J. I., Keenan, K., & Winslow, E. B. (1996). Early risk factors and pathways in the development of early disruptive behavior problems. *Development and Psychopathology, 8,* 679–699.

Snyder, J., Edwards, P., McGraw, K., Kilgore, K., & Holton, A. (1994). Escalation and reinforcement in mother–child conflict: Social processes associated with the development of physical aggression. *Development and Psychopathology, 6,* 305–321.

Snyder, J., West, L., Stockemer, V., Givens, S., & Almquist-Parks, L. (1996). A social learning model of peer choice in the natural environment. *Journal of Applied Developmental Psychology, 17,* 215–237.

Spanier, G. B. (1976). Measuring dyadic adjustment: New scales for assessing the quality of marriage and similar dyads. *Journal of Marriage and the Family, 38,* 15–28.

Spear, L. P. (2000a). Neurobehavioral changes in adolescence. *Current Directions in Psychological Science, 9,* 111–114.

Spear, L. P. (2000b). The adolescent brain and age-related behavioral manifestations. *Neuroscience and Biobehavioral Reviews, 24,* 417–463.

Spoth, R. L., Kavanagh, K., & Dishion, T. J. (2002). Family-centered preventive intervention science: Toward benefits to larger populations of children, youth, and families. In R. L. Spoth, K. Kavanagh, & T. J. Dishion (Eds.), Universal family-centered prevention strategies: Current findings and critical issues for public health impact [Special Issue]. *Prevention Science, 3,* 145–152.

Spoth, R. L., & Redmond, C. (1993). Identifying program preferences through conjoint analysis: Illustrative results from a parent sample. *American Journal of Health Promotion, 8,* 124–133.

Spoth, R. L., & Redmond, C. (1996). Illustrating a framework for rural prevention research: Project family studies of rural family participation and outcomes. In R. D. Peters & R. J. McMahon (Eds.), *Preventing childhood disorders, substance abuse, and delinquency* (pp. 299–328). Newbury Park, CA: Sage.

Stattin, H., & Magnusson, D. (1991). Stability and change in criminal behaviour up to age 30. *British Journal of Criminology, 31,* 327–346.

Steinberg, L. (1988). Reciprocal relation between parent–child distance and pubertal maturation. *Developmental Psychology, 24,* 122–128.

Stoolmiller, M. S. (1990). *Parent supervision, child unsupervised wandering, and child antisocial behavior: A latent growth curve analysis.* Unpublished doctoral dissertation, University of Oregon, Eugene.

Stoolmiller, M. (1994). Antisocial behavior, delinquent peer association and unsupervised wandering for boys: Growth and change from childhood to early adolescence. Multivariate *Behavioral Research, 29,* 263–288.

Stormshak, E. A., & Dishion, T. J. (2002). An ecological approach to child and family clinical and counseling psychology. *Clinical Child and Family Psychology Review*, 5(3), 197–215.

Stouthamer-Loeber, M., Loeber, R., Van Kammen, W. B., & Zhang, Q. (1995). Uninterrupted delinquent careers: The timing of parental help-seeking in juvenile court contact. *Studies on Crime and Crime Prevention*, 4, 236–251.

Sue, D. W., Bingham, R. P., Porche-Burke, L., & Vasquez, M. (1999). The diversification of psychology: A multicultural revolution. *American Psychologist*, 54(12), 1061–1069.

Sugai, G., Horner, R. H., & Sprague, J. R. (1999). Functional assessment-based behavior support planning: Research to practice to research. *Behavior Disorders*, 24, 253–257.

Sullivan, H. S. (1953). *The interpersonal theory of psychiatry.* New York: Norton.

Szapocznik, J., & Kurtines, W. M. (1989). *Breakthroughs in family therapy with drug-abusing and problem youth.* New York: Springer.

Szapocznik, J., Kurtines, W. M., & Fernandez, T. (1980). Bicultural involvement and adjustment in Hispanic American youths. *International Journal of Intercultural Relations*, 4, 353–366.

Szapocznik, J., Kurtines, W. Santisteban, D. A., Pantin, H., Scopetta, M., Mancilla, Y., Aisenberg, S., McIntosh, S., Perez-Vidal, A., & Coatsworth, J. D. (1997). The evolution of structural ecosystemic theory for working with Latino families. In J. G. Garcia & M. C. Zea (Eds.), *Psychological interventions and research with Latino populations* (pp. 160–190). Needham Heights, MA: Allyn & Bacon.

Szapocznik, J., Perez-Vidal, A., Brickman, A. L., Foote, F. H., Santisteban, D., & Hervis, O. (1988). Engaging adolescent drug abusers and their families in treatment: A strategic structural systems approach. *Journal of Consulting and Clinical Psychology*, 56(4), 552–557.

Szapocznik, J., & Williams, R. A. (2000). Brief strategic family therapy: Twenty-five years of interplay among theory, research, and practice in adolescent behavior problems and drug abuse. *Clinical Child and Family Psychology Review*, 3, 117–134.

Taylor, T. K., & Biglan, A. (1998). Behavioral family interventions for improving child-rearing: A review of the literature for clinicians and policy makers. *Clinical Child and Family Psychology Review*, 1, 41–60.

Telch, M. J., Killen, J. D., McAlister, A. L., Perry, C. L., & Maccoby, N. (1982). Long-term follow-up of a pilot project on smoking prevention with adolescents. *Journal of Behavior Medicine*, 5, 1–7.

Trickett, E. J., & Birman, D. (1989). Taking ecology seriously: A community development approach to individually based preventive interventions in schools: In L. A. Bond & B. E. Compas (Eds.), *Primary prevention and promotion in the schools: Primary prevention of psychopathology* (Vol. 12, pp. 361–390). Newbury Park, CA: Sage.

Visher, E. B., & Visher, J. S. (1979). *Stepfamilies: A guide to working with stepparents and stepchildren.* New York: Brunner/Mazel.

Vitaro, F., Gendreau, P. L., Tremblay, R. E., & Oligny, P. (1998). Reactive and proactive aggression differentially predict later conduct problems. *Journal of Child Psychiatry and Psychology*, 39, 377–385.

Walker, H. M., Colvin, G., & Ramsey, E. (1995). *Antisocial behavior in school: Strategies and best practices.* Pacific Grove, CA: Brooks/Cole.

Walker, H. M., & Severson, H. H. (1991). *Systematic screening for behavior disorders: Training manual.* Longmont, CO: Sopris West.

Walsh, S. M. (1999). *Gender differences in the protective effects of planning orientation on the sexual activity and deviant peer influence of at-risk adolescents.* Unpublished doctoral dissertation, University of Oregon, Eugene.

Weber, F. D. (1998). *The dose–effect relationship in family therapy for conduct disordered youth.* Unpublished doctoral dissertation, University of Oregon, Eugene.

Webster-Stratton, C. (1984). Randomized trial of two parent-training programs for families with conduct-disordered children. *Journal of Consulting and Clinical Psychology, 52,* 666–678.

Webster-Stratton, C. (1990). Long-term follow-up of families with young conduct problem children: From preschool to grade school. *Journal of Clinical Child Psychology, 19,* 144–149.

Webster-Stratton, C. (1992). Individually administered videotape parent training: "Who benefits?" *Cognitive Therapy and Research, 16,* 31–52.

Webster-Stratton, C., & Herbert, M. (1993). "What really happens in parent training?" *Behavior Modification, 17*(4), 407–456.

Webster-Stratton, C., Kolpacoff, M., & Hollingsworth, T. (1988). Self-administered videotape therapy for families with conduct-problem children: Comparison with two cost-effective treatments and a control group. *Journal of Consulting and Clinical Psychology, 56,* 558–566.

Weiss, B., Catron, T., Harris, V., & Phung, T. M. (1999). The effectiveness of traditional child psychotherapy. *Journal of Consulting and Clinical Psychology, 68*(6), 1094–1101.

Weiss, R. L., Halford, W. K., & Kim. W. (1996). Managing marital therapy: Helping partners change. In V. B. van Hasslet & M. Hersen (Eds.), *Sourcebook of psychological treatment manuals for adult disorders* (pp. 489–537). New York: Plenum Press.

Weisz, J. R., Weiss, B., Hahn, S. S., Granger, D. A., & Morten, D. (1995). Effects of psychotherapy with children and adolescents revisited: A meta-analysis of treatment outcome studies. *Psychological Bulletin, 117,* 450–468.

Wills, T. A., Sandy, J. M., & Shinar, O. (1999). Cloninger's constructs related to substance use level and problems in late adolescence: A mediational model on self-control and coping motives. *Experimental and Clinical Psychopharmacology, 7*(2), 122–134.

Wills, T. A., Vaccaro, D., & McNamara, G. (1992). The role of life events, family support, and competence in adolescent substance use: A test of vulnerability and protective factors. *American Journal of Community Psychology, 20,* 349–374.

Wilson, D. W. (1980). *The natural selection of populations and communities.* Menlo Park, CA: Benjamin/Cummings.

Yamaguchi, K., & Kandel, D. B. (1985). On resolution of role incompatibility: A life event history analysis of family roles and marijuana use. *American Journal of Sociology, 90,* 1284–1325.

Index

DioNA